MILD TRAUMATIC BRAIN INJURY AND POSTCONCUSSION SYNDROME

OXFORD WORKSHOP SERIES:

AMERICAN ACADEMY OF CLINICAL NEUROPSYCHOLOGY

Series Editors

Greg J. Lamberty, *Editor-in-Chief*
Ida Sue Baron
Richard Kaplan
Sandra Koffler
Jerry Sweet

Volumes in the Series

Ethical Decision Making in Clinical Neuropsychology
Shane S. Bush

Mild Traumatic Brain Injury and Postconcussion Syndrome
Michael A. McCrea

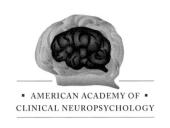

• AMERICAN ACADEMY OF •
CLINICAL NEUROPSYCHOLOGY

MILD TRAUMATIC BRAIN INJURY AND POSTCONCUSSION SYNDROME

The New Evidence Base for Diagnosis and Treatment

Michael A. McCrea

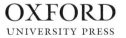

OXFORD WORKSHOP SERIES

OXFORD
UNIVERSITY PRESS

2008

OXFORD
UNIVERSITY PRESS

Oxford University Press, Inc., publishes works that further
Oxford University's objective of excellence
in research, scholarship, and education.

Oxford   New York
Auckland   Cape Town   Dar es Salaam   Hong Kong   Karachi
Kuala Lumpur   Madrid   Melbourne   Mexico City   Nairobi
New Delhi   Shanghai   Taipei   Toronto

With offices in
Argentina   Austria   Brazil   Chile   Czech Republic   France   Greece
Guatemala   Hungary   Italy   Japan   Poland   Portugal   Singapore
South Korea   Switzerland   Thailand   Turkey   Ukraine   Vietnam

Published by Oxford University Press, Inc.
198 Madison Avenue, New York, New York 10016

www.oup.com

Library of Congress Cataloging-in-Publication Data
McCrea, Michael, 1965–
Mild traumatic brain injury and post-concussion syndrome : the new
evidence base for diagnosis and treatment / Michael McCrea.
p. ; cm.—(Oxford workshop series)
Includes bibliographical references and index.
ISBN 978-0-19-532829-5
1. Brain damage.   2. Brain—Concussion.
[DNLM: 1. Brain Injuries.   2.   Post-Concussion Syndrome. WL 354 M4775m 2007]
I. American Academy of Clinical Neuropsychology.   II. Title.   III. Series.
RC387.5.M398 2007
616.8'0475—dc22   2007010728

7 9 8 6

Printed in the United States of America
on acid-free paper

Contents

Introduction

Mild traumatic brain injury (MTBI) has long been considered one of the most perplexing and challenging encounters for clinicians throughout the neurosciences. In most cases, neurosurgeons appropriately release MTBI patients from their care once it is clear that there are no medical emergencies in need of surgical intervention; neurologists are rightfully frustrated by how the symptoms and course of MTBI often do not conveniently fit into a plausible neurologic explanation; and factions within neuropsychology have forever debated whether neurologic or psychological factors are the basis for persistent problems after MTBI. For years, we have had difficulty coming to a consensus on even what to call these injuries—"concussion," "mild closed head injury," "mild head injury," and "mild traumatic brain injury" are often used interchangeably, sometimes within the same sentence. MTBI is the prevailing term adopted by the scientific community in recent years and is used throughout this text.

Our inability to answer one question, more than any other, is the nemesis that has hampered our understanding of this injury: *What is the true natural history of MTBI?* Clinicians in a variety of clinical and forensic settings are frequently asked to answer this question. Historically, science has fallen short in plotting the true natural history of MTBI. The existing literature indicates that most individuals reach a full recovery within three months of suffering an MTBI, but the rate of recovery is quite variable, and a small percentage of patients continue to report ongoing symptoms commonly characterized as postconcussion syndrome (PCS). For this subgroup with persistent symptoms, clinicians frequently face the challenge of trying to objectively measure the cognitive and symptomatic effects of injury and differentiating the neurologic or psychological factors that are contributing to the patient's persistent symptoms. Obviously, this differentiation is critical to prescribing appropriate treatment for the MTBI patient, the most effective form of which, unfortunately, has also historically not been well established. Challenges related to MTBI case definition, evaluation, and treatment have also confounded our measurement of eventual outcome associated with these injuries.

Thankfully, the science of MTBI has advanced more in the past decade than in the prior half century. In 1998, the Consensus Conference on Traumatic Brain Injury Rehabilitation, sponsored by the National Institutes of Health, identified 30 areas in need of additional research. A review of the literature now reflects that several studies have since been published and generated new knowledge on TBI epidemiology, effects, management, complications, rehabilitation, and outcome.[1] Researchers, including neuropsychologists, recently recognized many of the methodological flaws of traditional MTBI research (e.g., motor vehicle accident paradigms) and began to "think outside the box" to discover more innovative ways to study MTBI.[2] This new perspective has created a whole new platform for prospective MTBI research. As in all areas of medicine, MTBI research has also greatly benefited from technological advances in neuroradiologic, neurophysiologic, and biologic testing.

As a result, many recent breakthroughs have advanced our understanding of the biomechanics, neurophysiology, clinical presentation, and expected outcome associated with MTBI. Collectively, this body of work moves us closer to a more complete understanding of the true natural history of MTBI, which ideally should translate directly to evidence-based methods for clinical evaluation, management, and, ultimately, improved outcome. These new research findings also challenge traditional lines of thinking about MTBI by contrasting long-held assumptions with what the scientific base really shows.

One movement in MTBI research has been particularly fruitful over the past two decades. In the early 1980s, neuropsychologists were called upon to consult with sports medicine clinicians in evaluating the effects and recovery from concussion in collegiate and professional athletes. A core group of neuropsychologists quickly realized that the sports concussion assessment model not only provides direct benefit to the sports medicine community, but also creates a unique laboratory to advance our scientific understanding of the effects and recovery after MTBI in general. There has since been an explosion in sports concussion research, led predominantly by neuropsychologists, that has led to key findings that now provide the first evidence base to guide clinicians in the evaluation, interpretation, and treatment of MTBI and PCS.

This is perhaps the perfect point, up front and center, to declare that this text is not intended as another sports concussion book. Contrary to previous texts, this book focuses more on scientific updates that influence the clinical management of all MTBI and PCS, and less on sports-specific issues. You will find no discussion of which concussion grading scale is best, debate on return-to-play decision making, or instructions on how to develop a neuropsychological testing program for sports teams. Rather, the specific aim of this book is to, where appropriate, transfer findings from sports concussion research to our understanding of MTBI in general clinical practice.

To that end, the book provides a brief overview of the methodological advantages inherent to the sports concussion research model, followed by presentation of data from several recent large-scale, prospective studies applying standardized assessment methods, neuropsychological testing, and functional magnetic resonance imaging (fMRI) to investigate the natural history of MTBI. Special emphasis is placed on a review of innovative studies and key findings appearing in the MTBI literature over the past five years.

If MTBI has perplexed clinicians for years, the mere prospect of PCS has caused many to run and hide. PCS has been plagued by gaps in the MTBI research that leave questions about the syndrome's definition and accurate diagnosis, etiology, true incidence, clinical characteristics, expected outcome, and most effective options for treatment. The goal of this book is to provide an integrated, high-level review of emerging MTBI science over the past decade that ultimately helps clinicians reframe our understanding of PCS diagnosis and treatment.

The book follows a natural progression from the epidemiology to outcome associated with MTBI. It begins with a brief review of the broader scope of all-severity TBI, and then zeroes in on new, ground-breaking research findings specific to MTBI. The review is organized into the following four parts.

In part one, "The TBI Landscape," the range of traumatic brain injury (TBI) severity and defining injury characteristics is briefly reviewed, with special emphasis on the epidemiology, clinical significance, and public health implications of MTBI. Shortcomings of traditional MTBI research paradigms are addressed, and the advantages of new, innovative research models (e.g., sports concussion as MTBI laboratory) are highlighted. Part one also provides the foundation that frames later discussion of transferring recent findings from sports concussion research to MTBI in a general clinical setting and, ultimately, the diagnosis and treatment of PCS.

Part two, "Basic and Clinical Science of MTBI," presents findings from recent research on the biomechanics, neuropathology, and neurometabolic cascade associated with MTBI, not previously available from traditional MTBI research models. The utility of advanced neuroimaging methods in MTBI is discussed, and new data are reviewed that support the importance of assessment during the acute phase as the best method for establishing the diagnosis of MTBI and determining the proper course of early intervention, as prescribed by the World Health Organization's Collaborating Centre Task Force on Mild Traumatic Brain Injury.[3]

In part three, recent findings from prospective studies illustrating the natural history of MTBI are reviewed, including data that quantitatively plot the course of recovery in symptoms, cognitive functioning, and postural stability beginning within minutes of injury. The latest reports on neuropsychological recovery after MTBI are reviewed, and the influence of acute injury characteristics (e.g., unconsciousness, amnesia) on measuring severity of MTBI and subsequent recovery are illustrated based on the latest research. Recent studies on the sensitivity/specificity and incremental value of neuropsychological testing are reviewed, as well, including a comparison of effect sizes from neuropsychological studies of MTBI and other conditions known to cause cognitive dysfunction. The functional neuroimaging literature on neurophysiologic effects and recovery after MTBI are summarized. The age-old question of expected outcome after MTBI is addressed based on the latest empirical evidence, with a special section looking at the potential long-term effects of recurrent MTBI.

Part four, in keeping with the ultimate intention of this book, transfers findings from recent studies and nontraditional research platform (e.g., sports concussion) to the broader picture of the evaluation and treatment of MTBI in general clinical practice. Special emphasis is placed on the implications of those empirical findings reviewed throughout the book to our understanding of postconcussive syndrome (PCS). A thorough review is presented of various methodological issues that influence the epidemiologic and clinical study of PCS, and findings from recent studies are presented that shed new light on true incidence, etiology, and outcome associated with PCS. Psychological theories of PCS and proposed interventional models for treatment of PCS are discussed.

Every attempt has been made to provide key information in easily referenced tables and figures where appropriate throughout the book. Also, in keeping with the goal of providing researchers and clinicians with a boiled down capsule of key empirical findings, each part concludes with a summary of the top 10 conclusions or "take-home" points of greatest importance.

Certain limitations of this book also deserve acknowledgment. Like others in the collaborative series between Oxford University Press and the American Academy of Clinical Neuropsychology, this text is intended as a high-level overview of the topic, in this case MTBI, but cannot accomplish an exhaustive review of every study in each respective area (e.g., neuropsychological testing, neuroimaging) of the literature. My hope is that this text will provide the reader with a valuable shelf reference that effectively summarizes the scientific literature on MTBI and establishes an evidence base to drive "best practice" in the evaluation and management of MTBI and PCS. I have wished for such a resource for several years, and I hope that this book equally fills a void in your library of clinical resources.

Continuing Education Credit

To access the book's Continuing Education component, visit
http://theaacn.org/ce/book_series

Author's Workshop Materials

To download materials from the author's workshop presentation, such as PowerPoints, visit
www.oup.com/us/companion.websites/9780195328295

References

1. Ragnarsson KT. Traumatic brain injury research since the 1998 NIH Consensus Conference: accomplishments and unmet goals. *J Head Trauma Rehabil* 2006;21(5):379–87.

2. Barth JT, Freeman JR, Winters JE. Management of sports-related concussions. *Dent Clin North Am* 2000;44(1):67–83.

3. Carroll LJ, Cassidy JD, Holm L, Kraus J, Coronado VG. Methodological issues and research recommendations for mild traumatic brain injury: the WHO Collaborating Centre Task Force on Mild Traumatic Brain Injury. *J Rehabil Med* 2004(43 suppl):113–25.

Acknowledgments

This book would not have been possible without the help and support of many people. In reality, you could say that this book has been a work in progress for the past several years. During that time, I have been fortunate enough to work with an incredible team of collaborators from neurosurgery, neurology, neuropsychology, epidemiology, athletic training, and physiatry—all of whom now constitute our clinical research group known as the Concussion Research Consortium. I owe James Kelly, MD, and Christopher Randolph, PhD, an enormous debt of gratitude for introducing me to the world of traumatic brain injury, both clinically and scientifically, during my fellowship training more than a decade ago. My work with Kevin Guskiewicz, PhD, ATC, a world leader in sports concussion research, has proven to be a perfect partnership that has generated much of the work reviewed in this book. Thomas Hammeke, PhD, took the baton from Drs. Kelly and Randolph and has provided me with invaluable mentorship that paved the way for projects like this book. William Barr, PhD, has also been a key collaborator in much of the work presented herein, as well as a great friend. The encouragement of my partners in clinical practice (Drs. Gina Rehkemper, Pamela McMurray, Matthew Powell, and Sarah Sengstock) and support of administration at my host institution (Waukesha Memorial Hospital, ProHealth Care) kept this project on track when other demands were also calling. Obviously, our research team is most grateful to all those researchers whose work paved the way for this book and the thousands of subjects that have participated in our research over the years that advanced the science of MTBI, which now benefits all in the broader neurosciences.

Finally, the unending support of my wife, Ann Marie, my daughters, Grace and Elena, and my entire family has always been incredible. That was perhaps never more apparent than during the writing of this book, much of which took place on their watch. I am fortunate to have the best of both worlds, surrounded by colleagues I cherish, with an even richer life at home.

PART ONE

THE TBI LANDSCAPE

I

Epidemiology and Impact of Traumatic Brain Injury

In order to eventually put mild traumatic brain injury (MTBI) into proper perspective, it is important to first paint the broader picture of the significance of all-severity traumatic brain injury (TBI). TBI is one of the most significant public health problems facing the United States and other industrialized countries around the world. Every year, TBI is a leading cause of death and disability among young people.[1] National estimates of TBI in the United States range anywhere from 1.4 million[1] to 3 million[2] brain injuries per year, depending on the study and methods used to define and include cases. In 2003, there were an estimated 1,224,000 hospital emergency department visits, 290,000 hospitalizations, and 51,000 deaths resulting from TBI,[3] all of which sum to a total of 1,565,000 hospital-treated TBIs that year.

Given changes in hospitalization patterns over the past two decades, fewer and fewer mild and moderate TBI patients are hospitalized, with more triaged in the emergency department or treated in ambulatory/outpatient settings, so the true incidence of all-severity TBI is severely underestimated. As a result, the real extent of emergency department and ambulatory or outpatient diagnosis and treatment of brain injury remains unclear.[4] It has long been held that a significant percentage of individuals with milder brain injuries seek no medical attention after their injury, and therefore are not captured in epidemiologic studies that depend on hospital-based data. Some studies, for example, include only patients hospitalized, while others include patients treated and released from the hospital emergency department. Years ago, Fife[5] estimated that only 16 percent of all head injuries resulted in an admission to a hospital. Other reports have suggested that perhaps as many as 25 percent of all TBIs have no contact with the health care system at any level. Given the limitations of existing data sets and the complications in capturing any and all reportable incidents of TBI, most agree that published estimates significantly underrepresent the true incidence and prevalence of TBI. Furthermore, it is likely that a larger proportion of cases unaccounted for fall at the milder end of the TBI severity continuum, thereby drastically underestimating the prevalence of MTBI in particular.

Who Is at Risk?

Several studies indicate that the youngest and oldest members of a population are at greatest risk of TBI. Age-specific rates show a bimodal distribution, with highest risk in very young persons and people more than 64 years of age. Nearly half a million children in the United States are affected by TBI each year, making it one of the most serious public health problems affecting young people.[6] Some studies of TBI occurrence in the U.S. report that individuals 15–24 years old are at the highest risk, while several studies have also reported higher TBI rates among young children (0–4 years old).[3] In fact, TBI is the single leading cause of death and disability in the pediatric age group.[7]

While the epidemiology and significance of brain injury in childhood and adolescence have been recognized for some time, new awareness of the impact of head injury in older adults has more recently emerged. Recent reviews report that adults 75 or more years of age have the highest rates of TBI-related hospitalization and death.[8] As many as 80,000 persons 65 or older are treated for TBI in hospital emergency departments each year, and up to 75 percent of these visits result in hospitalization.[8] In contrast to younger victims, among older victims falls are more commonly the cause of injury, and motor vehicle crashes are second. Advanced age has also been associated with poorer outcome after TBI. Older individuals are reportedly at greater risk of dying in the hospital, requiring health care assistance after hospitalization, and being discharged from the hospital to a long-term care or rehabilitation facility.[1] In the older population, both age and use of oral anticoagulation increase the risk of mortality after TBI.[9]

Gender is also a factor affecting an individual's risk of TBI. All published studies report higher occurrence of TBI among men than among women. Age-adjusted TBI rates for males have been found to be approximately twice that of females (91.9 vs. 47.7/100,000, respectively).[10] The bimodal age distribution of TBI pertains to both males and females, with younger (younger than 15) and older people at greatest risk (older than 65),[10] regardless of gender.

Higher incidence of TBI has been reported in minorities than in whites, but this finding is debated based on inconsistencies across study methodologies, mechanism for case recording, and the interaction between race and other factors tied to TBI risk (e.g., socioeconomic factors).

A U.S. epidemiologic study[10] reported that TBI-related hospital discharge rates were highest for American Indians/Alaskan Natives (75.3 per 100,000 population) and blacks (74.4 per 100,000). Specifically, black males and Native Americans had the highest rates of TBI attributable to assault, which was four times the rate for white males. Among children, higher death and hospitalization rates have been reported among blacks than among whites for TBI resulting from motor vehicle accidents.

Several studies have reported higher TBI rates among individuals at the lowest socioeconomic levels.[11,12] As noted, however, an interaction of several factors tied to socioeconomic status (e.g., race/ethnicity, exposure to violent crime, housing) complicates interpretation of the direct impact of socioeconomic factors alone on TBI risk.

In terms of lifestyle factors, substance abusers are at significantly higher risk of TBI. This factor, however, is confounded by a generally higher risk for all external causes of injury (TBI and otherwise) resulting from alcohol and drug abuse, including motor vehicle crashes, assaults, and falls. Because of population substance use patterns, alcohol is the main culprit more often than other illicit drugs. As many as half of all TBI patients treated in hospital emergency departments have a positive blood alcohol concentration, and the majority of those have blood alcohol concentration levels above the legal limit.[4] Although there is assumed elevated risk for TBI with other drug use, there are fewer empirical data available to make this connection.

Motor vehicle crashes have consistently been cited as the most common cause of TBI, accounting for 40–60 percent of all TBIs annually.[4] All forms of transportation, however, are common causes of TBI, including motorcycle crashes, bicycle accidents, and pedestrian injuries. The other leading causes of TBI are falls, assaults, and sports, with varied frequency across the life span.

Societal Impact of TBI

Injury of any type is one of the leading causes of mortality, and the leading cause of death among people 1 to 45 years of age. TBI is among the most prevalent and serious of all traumatic injuries: about 40 percent of trauma fatalities in the United States are due to brain injury.[4] Worldwide, at least 10 million TBIs serious enough to result in death or hospitalization occur annually,[13] and an estimated 57 million people in the world have been hospitalized for TBI. Each year, there are an estimated 50,000–100,000 TBI-related deaths in the United Sates. This figure has remained relatively stable over several years and is similar to rates reported in other parts of the world.

There is also no question that TBI imposes substantial demands on the U.S. health care system.[14] When we look at the full spectrum of central nervous system disorders, TBI has the third highest hospital discharge rate (86.6 discharges per 100,000 population), behind only stroke and schizophrenic disorders.[15] Pediatric TBI itself is a substantial contributor to health resource burden in the United States, with estimated hospital charges of more than $1 billion per year.[16] As far back as 1991, the total cost of brain injury in the United States was estimated at $48.3 billion annually, with hospitalization accounting for $31.7 billion and TBI-related fatalities costing the nation $16.6 billion each year.[17] Based on epidemiologic data, inflation, and rising health care costs, it seems safe to assume that the cost of TBI is in the order of $100 billion in today's dollars.

With advances in modern medicine, more people are surviving TBI than ever before. An estimated 5.3 million Americans are living with significant disabilities resulting from prior TBI that significantly complicate their return to a full and productive life,[18] which is roughly 1 in every 10 of the 54 million Americans with disability. Each year, at least 20 percent of individuals hospitalized for treatment of TBI leave the hospital with moderate to severe disabilities.[10] In 2000, Krause[4] estimated nearly 100,000 people in the United States acquired new disabilities from mild, moderate or severe TBI. Brain injury accounts for more lost productivity among Americans than any other form of injury. To put into perspective, it is estimated that the percentage (15.7 percent) of injury-related productivity loss attributed to TBI is 14 times that associated with spinal cord injury.[19]

Conclusion

Without question, TBI is one of the greatest public health problems in the United States and worldwide, whether measured in terms of true incidence, morbidity and mortality, economic burden, or the resulting impact on the lives of TBI victims and their families. This chapter has strategically distinguished mild from moderate and severe TBI, thereby providing a framework for our focused discussion of the science specific to MTBI throughout the remainder of the book.

2

Zeroing In on MTBI:
Epidemiology and Impact

Attention turns now from the broader landscape of all-severity TBI to more narrowly focus on MTBI. Despite the severity rating as "mild," MTBI packs a powerful punch both in sheer volume of injuries and in societal impact. In 2003, the Centers for Disease Control and Prevention (CDC) presented to the U.S. Congress a report describing MTBI as a "silent epidemic,"[20] based on concerns that the true incidence and ultimate public health impact of MTBI are severely underestimated. All aspects of MTBI, from epidemiology to diagnosis, treatment, and outcome, are of increasing importance to health care professionals and researchers. In the last five years, both the CDC and the World Health Organization (WHO) have published reports to elevate awareness of the public health impact of MTBI in the minds of policy makers at both the state and federal level.

It is estimated that 70–90 percent of all treated TBIs are mild in severity based on traditional case definitions and acute injury characteristic criteria,[21] with most reported estimates in the order of 85 percent.[22] In a 2004 report, the WHO Collaborating Centre Task Force on Mild Traumatic Brain Injury cited the incidence of hospital-treated MTBI as be 100–300/100,000 population.[23] The investigators point out, however, that this figure and others in the literature may underrepresent the true incidence of MTBI because of variable case definitions and heterogeneous methods. Add to these methodological issues the fact that many cases of MTBI have no hospital contact, and the true population-based rate of MTBI is probably more on the order of 500/100,000 population.

In 2005, Bazarian et al.[22] reported the incidence of emergency department visits for MTBI to be 503/100,000, which computes to approximately 1.4 million emergency department visits for MTBI each year in the United States. In sum, MTBI is estimated to account for just more than 1 percent of all hospital emergency department visits per year in the United States. Of all patients with emergency department visits for MTBI, fewer than 10 percent are admitted to the hospital.[22] In a medium-sized community hospital with approximately 50,000 emergency department visits per year, that equates to roughly 10 MTBI-related encounters per week, 9 of whom will be treated and released from the emergency department, often with variable recommendations for medical follow-up.

The higher population-based incidence rate reported by Bazarian et al.[22] relative to other studies is possibly attributable to a multitude of factors, including a generally increasing rate of hospital emergency department contacts for all health care, underestimation of true TBI incidence in prior studies, and expansion of the International Classification of Diseases, ninth revision (ICD-9) codes included in the study's case definition. In keeping with the CDC administrative definition of MTBI, the study by Bazarian et al. included a new code, "head injury, unspecified," which accounted for 73 percent of all MTBI cases captured in the study (356/100,000 population). In contrast, "concussion" was the formal diagnosis in just more than 20 percent of all MTBI cases, with a small percentage of skull fracture and unspecified intracranial injury diagnoses.

The impact of diagnostic coding accuracy on determining the true incidence of MTBI has also been addressed by Bazarian et al.[24] In a study of more than 35,000 patients presenting to an urban academic medical center emergency department, 1.47 percent ($n = 516$) met the clinical criteria for diagnosis of MTBI, while twice as many ($n = 1,000$) were assigned one or more ICD-9 codes for MTBI. Specifically, 45 percent of patients coded as "head injury, unspecified" did not meet the clinical definition of MTBI. These findings underscore the need for thorough clinical evaluation to establish the diagnosis of MTBI based on biomechanics, acute injury characteristics, and course of symptoms, while also highlighting the problems inherent to epidemiologic studies based on retrospective review of less reliable diagnostic codes chiefly intended for administrative and billing purposes.

Most believe that the inclusion of "head injury, unspecified" in the case definition of MTBI likely overestimates the true incidence of MTBI. In the other direction, however, MTBI incidence is likely underestimated by the fact that a large percentage of MTBI patients have no contact with a hospital emergency department or, for that matter, any medical professional. Collectively, epidemiologic data seem to converge on a true incidence rate of MTBI in the order of 500/100,000 population, considering hospital-based studies and estimates of MTBI patients who seek no hospital-based treatment. Regardless of setting, these estimates quickly turn into real numbers. At the community-based hospital where I practice, with a population base of approximately 400,000, our emergency department sees anywhere from 1,500 to 2,000 MTBI patients per year.

Who Is at Risk of MTBI?

As in the case of all-severity TBI, higher rates of MTBI are reported among young males and minorities. Bazarian et al.,[22] for instance, reported MTBI incidence in children younger than 5 (1,115/100,000 population) to be more than double that of the non-age-adjusted rate (503/100,000). In general, the highest incidence rates of MTBI were observed in people younger than 24 and older than 74, similar to the data on the risk of all-severity TBI. Falls, motor vehicle crashes, cycling accidents, assaults, and other accidents are the most common causes of MTBI, with varied distribution across the age spectrum. For instance, falls account for the largest percentage of MTBI among the very young (younger than 5) and the elderly (older than 75). During the life span when people do their most driving, motor vehicle crashes are the most common cause of MTBI. Sports and recreation are a major cause of MTBI in adolescents and young adults, which is outlined in greater detail later in part one.

Economic and Societal Impact of MTBI

In 2003, the CDC concluded that MTBI is a major public health problem, the magnitude and impact of which are underestimated by current injury surveillance systems. [20] Although data from prospective hospital-based MTBI studies are limited, it is estimated that lost productivity after MTBI accounts for the largest component of the economic costs of brain trauma each year in the United States. The total economic effects and health care utilization associated with MTBI are substantial. While the intensity of care is less than in moderate and severe TBI (e.g., no intensive care, surgery, or lengthy hospitalization), the cost equation is balanced by sheer volume, especially when considering that 70–90 percent of all TBI fall into the mild category.

Analyzing U.S. TBI incidence and cost data from 1985, Max et al.[25] estimated that MTBI accounted for $16.5 billion (44 percent) of the estimated total lifetime cost ($37.8 billion) of TBIs that year. In 2001, the CDC updated these estimates using incidence data from 1995 and adjusting for inflation to yield an estimated total cost of $56 billion, $16.7 billion of which was associated with MTBI.[26] Both reports qualify their findings by suggesting that these figures underestimate the true economic burden that MTBI poses on the United States due to several factors, including the following:

- The totals do not include MTBIs treated and released from the emergency department or those who seek treatment in other nonhospital medical care settings (e.g., physician's office), and excludes those who seek no medical contact after MTBI.
- Costs of lost productivity and diminished quality of life are not incorporated into these totals.
- Indirect costs borne by family and others who care for the MTBI patient are not included.

Unfortunately, there are essentially no studies that provide estimates of the cost of MTBI in today's dollars. Considering that only about 10 percent of MTBI patients are ever hospitalized, there is no question that published figures underestimate the true economic impact of MTBI, whether measured in yesterday's or today's dollars.

Beyond health care utilization costs, even less is known about lost work time and productivity in the overwhelming majority of MTBI patients who are not hospitalized or seek no medical attention after MTBI and are therefore not captured at all in hospital-based studies of MTBI incidence and outcome. While it is well established that MTBI results in physical, cognitive, psychological, and social dysfunction that results in significant disability and lost productivity for a period of time after injury, few studies have quantified the impact of MTBI.

Boake et al.[27] reported that MTBI patients were comparable to general trauma patients in duration of work absence and problems reported after returning to work. Specifically, this study demonstrated that most MTBI patients who were treated and released from the hospital emergency department did not return to work until one to three months after injury. In the

MTBI patients, there was essentially no difference in rates of return to work for those that were treated and released from the emergency department (46 percent working at one month, 66 percent at three months, and 68 percent at six months) versus those who were hospitalized (39 percent working at one months, 62 percent at three months, and 71 percent at six months) after their injury. These figures are similar to those previously reported by Rimel et al.[28] and Dikmen et al.[29] Other studies with longer term follow-up have also shown the rate of return to work after MTBI to increase to upward of 85 percent between six months and two years postinjury.[29] A somewhat surprising finding was that patients employed in more cognitively demanding jobs (e.g., professional, technical, managerial) tended to return to work earlier than those working in jobs historically thought to be less vulnerable to the cognitive and other effects of MTBI (e.g., unskilled labor). Those individuals who were unemployed at the time of their TBI were also the least likely to return to work within six months of their injury (41 percent).

Conclusion

While there is no question that MTBI poses a significant public health problem in the United States and around the world, further study is required to precisely determine the public health impact of MTBI in terms of health care resource utilization, economic costs, lost productivity (in both inability to return to work and reduced capacity on the job), and societal burden.

3

Challenges in Defining and Diagnosing MTBI

It is now widely recognized that one of the great challenges facing clinicians in the diagnosis of MTBI is establishing a minimum threshold for injury and classifying the gradient of acute TBI injury severity along the traditional continuum from mild to moderate to severe. Ultimately, accurate diagnosis of injury severity would both drive injury management techniques during the acute postinjury phase and be predictive of recovery and outcome further out from injury. A growing body of literature, however, suggests that while these tenets may apply in moderate to severe forms of TBI, they do not map onto MTBI. In fact, the body of work on MTBI over the past decade suggests that MTBI may be a different animal all together from moderate and severe TBI (summarized in table 3.1).[30] These important distinctions that place MTBI in a category by itself set the stage for reframing our understanding of MTBI and our approach to diagnosis and treatment of postconcussion syndrome (PCS), which are the driving forces behind this book.

Conventional wisdom tells us that accurate injury detection and diagnosis of TBI will result in improved injury management and treatment, both of which will ultimately reduce mortality and enhance outcome following TBI. The first step in that process relates to recognizing and properly classifying TBI at all severity levels, which has proven to be an imperfect science and work in progress for years. Again, one size does not fit all in the case of TBI. That is, a classification system or injury grading scale that proves to be diagnostically accurate and predictive of outcome following moderate and severe TBI may be of limited utility in MTBI.

Numerous systems have been developed over the years to classify TBI severity along a continuum from mild to moderate to severe.[31] Some injury

Table 3.1 Key Distinctions Between Mild and Moderate/Severe TBI

	MODERATE AND SEVERE	MILD TBI
Definitions	Consistently anchored in injury mechanics, acute injury characteristics; consistent criteria across studies	Dependent upon symptoms; varied definitions across injury classification systems and empirical studies
Acute Injury Characteristics (e.g., LOC, PTA, focal neurologic deficits)	Often clearly present and documented; drivers of critical care management; strongest predictors or long-term outcome	Varied emphasis on presence and duration of LOC, PTA, mental status abnormalities, and constellation of symptoms; limited correlation with outcome
Classification Systems, Tools	Tried and true methods for classifying injury severity; strong history of GCS validity in grading injury severity and correlation with outcome	Traditional scales (e.g., GCS) of limited utility due to ceiling effect and limited sensitivity; GCS not initially intended for classification of MTBI; minimal penetration of any specific tool for standardized assessment of MTBI
Neuroimaging Studies	Imaging studies of critical diagnostic importance to identifying neurosurgical emergencies; significant advances in both structural and functional neuroimaging of moderate and severe TBI, correlated with clinical measures and outcome	In a clinical setting, neuroimaging negative and equivocal in overwhelming majority of cases, essentially by definition of MTBI; lack of "objective findings" restricts the medical legitimacy of MTBI; some indication that "complicated MTBI" with structural injury (and abnormal imaging) distinct from "uncomplicated MTBI" with no structural injury

Natural History of Injury, Recovery	Well defined and empirically delineated	Not well understood; limited to no consensus
Outcome	Injury severity, based on acute injury characteristics, the strongest predictor of recovery and outcome, with exceptions confounded by noninjury factors	Most often predicted by noninjury-related factors, e.g., premorbid psychosocial issues, psychological comorbidities, postinjury stressors, substance abuse, litigation
Persistent Disability	More clearly attributed to the severity, functional neuroanatomy of injury, and resulting impairments in most cases	Debated as to whether due to neurologic vs. psychological factors; true epidemiology, etiology of postconcussion syndrome unclear

GCS, Glasgow Coma Scale; LOC, loss of consciousness; PTA, posttraumatic amnesia.

Table 3.2 Glasgow Coma Scale (GCS)

Motor	6	Obeys verbal commands
	5	Localizes to noxious stimuli
	4	Normal flexion to noxious stimuli
	3	Abnormal flexion to noxious stimuli (decorticate posturing)
	2	Extension to noxious stimuli (decerebrate posturing)
	1	No response to noxious stimuli
Verbal	5	Fully oriented and converses
	4	Disoriented and converses
	3	Voices appropriate words
	2	Makes incomprehensible sounds
	1	No vocalization
Eye Opening	4	Opens eyes spontaneously
	3	Opens eyes to verbal commands
	2	Opens eyes to noxious stimuli
	1	No eye opening

Maximum GCS score = 15; minimum GCS score = 3
From Teasdale G, Jennett B. Assessment of coma and impaired consciousness; A practical scale. *Lancet* 1974; 2.

classification systems break down these broad categories even further and suggest several points of classification. In nearly all classification systems, TBI severity is graded based on acute injury characteristics. Historically, presence and duration of unconsciousness and amnesia have been the main points of distinction along the gradient of TBI severity, but these phenomena have been demonstrated to have less significance in predicting outcome after MTBI.

The Glasgow Coma Scale (GCS)[32] is far and away the most recognized and widely used method for grading TBI severity. The GCS assesses gross neurologic status across three core areas of motor function, verbal responding, and the patient's ability to open the eyes voluntarily or in response to external commands and stimuli, as outlined in table 3.2. The most basic approach to grading TBI severity is based solely on GCS score, with a range between 3 and 15 out of 15 (see table 3.3).

Table 3.3 Glasgow Coma Scale (GCS) TBI Severity Classification System

TBI SEVERITY	GCS SCORE
Mild	13–15
Moderate	8–12
Severe	3–9

From Jennett and Teasdale.[32]

Because the GCS was originally designed to assess a patient's level of consciousness, in either a prehospital or acute critical care environment, the scale has its greater natural application to classifying more severe forms of TBI that involve brief or extended unconsciousness or at least a gross alteration in level of consciousness. There has been debate about the predictive value of GCS scores obtained at a trauma scene or upon arrival at the hospital emergency department, which also has significant implications for clinical decision making during the triage phase. One study indicated that field GCS scores are highly predictive of arrival GCS scores and that both scores are associated with outcome from TBI.[33] Specifically, a change in GCS score from field to arrival was highly predictive of outcome.

Scales such as the GCS that depend largely on criteria susceptible only to more severe forms of neurologic dysfunction have inherent limitations when used to assess and classify more subtle neurologic conditions, including MTBI. By most traditional definitions, MTBI is classified based on a GCS score of 13–15. In reality, the overwhelming majority of patients treated and released from hospital emergency departments obtain the maximum score of 15 on the GCS. Consequently, there is a significant ceiling effect on the scale when applied in more mild forms of injury. That is, a score of 15 is sometimes interpreted as a completely normal neurologic status, free of any and all impairments that might be associated with TBI. It is well established, however, that the GCS is not sensitive to the defining characteristics of MTBI, namely common symptoms (e.g., headache, dizziness, nausea, sensitivity to light and noise) or alterations in mental status (e.g., confusion, disorientation, amnesia, poor concentration).

A general conclusion drawn by many in a clinical setting is that the GCS and similar scales have great value in the diagnosis of neurosurgical emergencies that require immediate triage, but have limited utility and sensitivity in the detection of MTBI. As a result, relying solely on these scales and their core criteria runs the risk of missing key diagnostic signs and symptoms not referenced by the scale, and ultimately underdiagnosing MTBI.

Defining MTBI: Looking Beyond GCS

Based on the distinctions between mild and moderate/severe TBI, it is widely recognized that a unique approach is required to operationally define MTBI. In response to the limitations inherent to traditional methods, several injury classification systems have been developed to go beyond GCS score or acute injury characteristics and incorporate chief signs and symptoms in defining MTBI.

Ommaya and Gennarelli[34] defined *cerebral concussion* as

> a graded set of clinical syndromes following head injury wherein increasing severity of disturbance in level and content of consciousness is caused by mechanically induced strains affecting the brain in a centripetal sequence of disruptive effect on brain function and structure.

These researchers offered a classification of the grades of concussion severity that considered multiple indicators from confusion to amnesia and unconsciousness (see table 3.4).

From the earlier work by Ommaya and Gennarelli, several scales have been developed to define and grade the severity of MTBI. The use of multiple severity indicators is intended to improve the sensitivity in the detection of MTBI, while also taking into consideration traditional acute injury characteristics that have been presumed to predict outcome following mild and moderate brain injury. Despite their limited utility in MTBI, loss of consciousness and posttraumatic amnesia (PTA) remain the most common injury characteristics referenced in most classification symptoms. Table 3.5 provides a matrix of criteria for the classification of mild, moderate, and severe TBI based on GCS and a combination of the total duration of unconsciousness and PTA.

An innovative system offered by Stein[31] expands beyond the classic mild-moderate-severe categorization of TBI severity and combines both GCS and acute injury characteristics, as described in table 3.6.

Table 3.4 Ommaya and Gennarelli Classification System for Grading Severity of Cerebral Concussion

SEVERITY GRADE	ALTERATION IN MENTAL STATUS	CHARACTERISTICS	HYPOTHESIZED PATHOPHYSIOLOGY
I	Confusion	Normal consciousness without amnesia	Cortical-subcortical disconnection (CSD)
II	Confusion and amnesia	Normal consciousness with confusion and posttraumatic amnesia (PTA)	CSD; possible diencephalic disconnection
III	Confusion and amnesia	Normal consciousness with confusion, PTA and retrograde amnesia (RGA)	CSD plus diencephalic disconnection (CSDD)
IV	Coma (paralytic)	Confusion with PTA and RGA	CSDD plus mesencephalic disconnection (CSDMD)
V	Coma	Persistent vegetative state	CSDMD
VI	Death	Fatal injury	CSDMD

Adapted from Ommaya and Gennarelli[34] with permission.

Table 3.5 Multiple Severity Indicators of Traumatic Brain Injury

	SEVERITY CLASSIFICATION		
MEASURE	MILD	MODERATE	SEVERE
Glasgow Coma Scale	13–15	9–12	3–8
Loss of consciousness	< 20 minutes	20 minutes to 36 hours	> 36 hours
Posttraumatic amnesia	< 24 hours	1–7 days	> 7 days

Adapted from Stein.[31]

The natural extension of injury classification systems is an attempt to establish a case or administrative definition to guide clinicians in recognizing the signs and symptoms of MTBI, formulate an accurate diagnosis, and prescribe appropriate treatment. On the research side, consensus definitions also serve as the basis for inclusion/exclusion criteria for enrollment in MTBI study protocols. One of the most commonly cited case definitions of *mild* TBI came from the Mild Traumatic Brain Injury Committee of the Head Injury Interdisciplinary Special Interest Group of the American Congress of Rehabilitation Medicine (ACRM).[35] The ACRM requires just a single criteria of uncon-

Table 3.6 Expanded Head Injury Severity Scale

SEVERITY CATEGORY	GCS SCORE AND ACUTE INJURY CHARACTERISTICS
Minimal	GCS = 15; no loss of consciousness (LOC) or amnesia
Mild	GCS = 14; or 15 plus amnesia; or brief (< 5 minutes) LOC, or impaired alertness, memory
Moderate	GCS = 9–13 or LOC > 5 minutes, or focal neurologic deficit
Severe	GCS = 5–8
Critical	GCS = 3–4

Reprinted from Stein[31] with permission.

sciousness, amnesia, or any alteration in mental status for the diagnosis of MTBI (see Box 3.1).

Although there is a fair amount of overlap across systems, other definitions of MTBI have placed varied emphasis on acute injury characteristics and other signs and symptoms to establish a diagnosis. Boxes 3.2–3.4 summarize the operational definitions of MTBI developed by the CDC MTBI Work Group,[20] the WHO Collaborating Centre Task Force on MTBI,[36] and the Defense and Veterans Brain Injury Center Working Group on the Acute Management of MTBI in Military Operational Settings, respectively.

Several classification systems and grading scales have also been developed for the diagnosis and management of sport-related concussion. As is the case of general (non-sport-related) MTBI, there is significant overlap across sports concussion classification systems, with some variation in the emphasis placed

BOX 3.2 CDC Conceptual Definition of MTBI

A case of MTBI is an occurrence of injury to the head resulting from blunt trauma or acceleration or deceleration forces with one or more of the following conditions attributable to the head injury during the surveillance period:

- Any period of observed or self-reported transient confusion, disorientation, or impaired consciousness;
- Any period of observed or self-reported dysfunction of memory (amnesia) around the time of injury;
- Observed signs of other neurological or neuropsychological dysfunction, such as—
    - Seizures acutely following head injury;
    - Among infants and very young children: irritability, lethargy, or vomiting following head injury;
    - Symptoms among older children and adults such as headache, dizziness, irritability, fatigue, or poor concentration, when identified soon after injury, can be used to support the diagnosis of mild TBI, but cannot be used to make the diagnosis in the absence of loss of consciousness or altered consciousness. Further research may provide additional guidance in this area.
- Any period of observed or self-reported loss of consciousness lasting 30 minutes or less.

More severe brain injuries were excluded from the definition of MTBI and include one or more of the following conditions attributable to the injury:

- Loss of consciousness lasting longer than 30 minutes;
- Posttraumatic amnesia lasting longer than 24 hours;
- Penetrating craniocerebral injury.

Adapted from the Report to Congress on Mild Traumatic Brain Injury in the United States: Steps to Prevent a Serious Public Health Problem. Atlanta, GA: National Center for Injury Prevention and Control, Centers for Disease Control and Injury Prevention, 2003.[20]

BOX 3.3 WHO Collaborating Centre Task Force on Mild Traumatic Brain Injury Operational Definition of MTBI*

MTBI is an acute brain injury resulting from mechanical energy to the head from external forces.

Operational criteria for clinical identification include:

    a. 1 or more of the following:

        i. Confusion or disorientation

        ii. Loss of consciousness for 30 minutes or less

        iii. Posttraumatic amnesia for less than 24 hours

        iv. Other transient neurological abnormalities such as focal signs, seizure, intracranial lesion not requiring surgery

    b. Glasgow Coma Scale score of 13–15 after 30 minutes postinjury or later upon presentation for health care

    c. These manifestations of MTBI must not be:

        i. Due to drugs, alcohol, medication

        ii. Caused by other injuries or treatment for other injuries (e.g., systemic injuries, facial injuries, or intubation)

        iii. Caused by other problems (e.g., psychological trauma, language barrier, or coexisting medical conditions)

        iv. Caused by penetrating craniocerebral injury

*WHO definition derived from ACRM and CDC definitions of MTBI.

Adapted from Holm et al.[37]

---

on certain injury severity indicators. Boxes 3.5 and 3.6 present the definition of concussion offered by the American Academy of Neurology[38] and the Concussion in Sport Group.[39,40]

The Elusive MTBI Denominator: Implications

Pinpointing the true epidemiology of TBI is complicated by a number of factors, and nowhere is this more problematic than in the case of MTBI. First, most published information comes from state or federal databases and is

BOX 3.4 Defense and Veterans Brain Injury Center Working Group on the Acute Management of Mild TBI in Military Operational Setting: Screening and Operational Definition of MTBI

Screening for MTBI

Anyone exposed to or involved in a blast, fall, vehicle crash, or direct impact who becomes dazed or confused, even momentarily, should be further evaluated for a brain injury.

Operational Definition of MTBI

Mild TBI in military operational settings is defined as an injury to the brain resulting from an external force and/or acceleration/deceleration mechanism from an event such as a blast, fall, direct impact, or motor vehicle accident which causes an alteration in mental status typically resulting in the temporally related onset of symptoms such as: headache, nausea, vomiting, dizziness/balance problems, fatigue, trouble sleeping/sleep disturbances, drowsiness, sensitivity to light/noise, blurred vision, difficulty remembering, and/or difficulty concentrating.

Adapted from the Defense and Veterans Brain Injury Center Clinical Practice Guideline.[37]

BOX 3.5 American Academy of Neurology (AAN) Guidelines for Management of Sports Concussion

Concussion is a trauma-induced alteration in mental status that may or may not involve loss of consciousness. Confusion and amnesia are the hallmarks of concussion. The confusional episode and amnesia may occur immediately after the blow to the head or several minutes later. Features of concussion frequently observed:
- Vacant stare (befuddled facial expression)
- Delayed verbal and motor responses (slow to answer questions or follow instructions)

(continued)

- Confusion and inability to focus attention (easily distracted and unable to follow through with normal activities)
- Disorientation (walking in the wrong direction, unaware of time, date and place.)
- Slurred or incoherent speech (making disjointed or incomprehensible statements)
- Gross observable incoordination (stumbling, inability to walk tandem/straight line)
- Emotions out of proportion to circumstances (distraught, crying for no apparent reason)
- Memory deficits
- Any period of loss of consciousness (paralytic coma, unresponsiveness to arousal)

The AAN Practice Parameter presents the following grading scale arrived at by a consensus of experts who reviewed all existing scales, including the recommendations in the Colorado Medical Society Guidelines:
- Grade 1: Transient confusion, no loss of consciousness, concussion symptoms, or mental status abnormalities on examination resolve in less than 15 minutes.
- Grade 2: Transient confusion, no Loss of consciousness, concussion symptoms or mental status abnormalities on examination last *more* than 15 minutes.
- Grade 3: Any loss of consciousness, either brief (seconds) or prolonged (minutes)

Symptoms of concussion: headache, dizziness or vertigo, lack of awareness of surroundings, nausea or vomiting, persistent low grade headache, light-headedness, poor attention and concentration, memory dysfunction, fatigability, irritability and low frustration tolerance, intolerance of bright lights or difficulty focusing vision, intolerance of loud noises, sometimes ringing in the ears, anxiety and/or depressed mood, sleep disturbance

---

Adapted from Kelly and Rosenberg.[38]

BOX 3.6 Concussion in Sport Group (CISG) Definition of Concussion (Vienna and Prague Statements)

Vienna Statement (2001)

Concussion is defined as a complex pathophysiological process affecting the brain, induced by traumatic biomechanical forces. Several common features that incorporate clinical, pathological, and biomechanical injury constructs that may be utilized in defining the nature of a concussive head injury include:

- Concussion may be caused either by a direct blow to the head, face, neck or elsewhere on the body with an "impulsive" force transmitted to the head.
- Concussion typically results in the rapid onset of short-lived impairment of neurological function that resolves spontaneously.
- Concussion may result in neuropathological changes, but the acute clinical symptoms largely reflect a functional disturbance rather than structural injury.
- Concussion results in a graded set of clinical syndromes that may or may not involve loss of consciousness. Resolution of the clinical and cognitive symptoms typically follows a sequential course.
- Concussion is typically associated with grossly normal structural neuroimaging studies.

Prague Statement (2004)

The CISG expanded on the definition from the Vienna statement by adding a separate classification for simple and complex concussion, as follows:

- *Simple concussion*: A concussion that resolves without complication over 7–10 days
- *Complex concussion*: A concussion with persistent symptoms, specific sequelae (such as concussive convulsions), prolonged loss of consciousness (more than one minute), or prolonged cognitive impairments. Multiple or repeat concussions can also be classified as complex.

Adapted from Aubry et al.[39] and McCrory et al.[40]

therefore limited to hospitalized patients. This raises an important point made by Kraus and Chu[4] that, although the clinical literature has inherent value for the practitioner, the epidemiologic literature provides a broader and more accurate assessment of the occurrence, characteristics, and consequences of TBI. Furthermore, both clinical and epidemiologic studies apply different case definitions, inclusion/exclusion criteria, and other key methodologies that result in varied sampling, and consequently varied findings. Any variance to this first link in the chain of research then obviously confounds the findings that come from these studies, especially when attempting to clarify the true natural history of MTBI and expected outcomes.

While the ACRM and other MTBI case definitions provide a general framework for the clinician in diagnosing MTBI, these criteria have also been subject to debate and criticism. For instance, the ACRM criteria stipulate a clear upper limit that defines the border between mild and moderate TBI (based on maximum duration of loss of consciousness/PTA and GCS score) but have what most consider to be a much softer threshold on the lower end of injury definition. For example, some argue that an alteration in mental status or amnesia surrounding a traumatic incident is not necessarily specific to TBI and can sometimes result from other factors, including psychological stress from general trauma. The reality is that there is no litmus test or gold standard to establish the criteria of "a traumatically induced physiologic disruption of brain function," and more often than not, the diagnosis of MTBI is based on acute injury characteristics and presenting signs and symptoms. Therein lies the problem in that the symptoms used to diagnose MTBI and PCS are almost exclusively nonspecific to MTBI and have rather high base rates in the normal, non-head-injured general population, particularly those exposed to general trauma without any occurrence of TBI.[41] This issue of nonspecificity of symptoms is discussed further in part four with specific relevance to PCS.

The implications for precisely pinpointing "the denominator" (i.e., the true incidence and prevalence of MTBI) are significant, both in a clinical setting and in applied research. Intellectual debate among experts on the definition of MTBI constantly volleys back and forth between arguments that certain criteria may result in the overinclusion or underreporting of MTBI.

In a clinical setting, the immediate issue of injury definition threshold relates to properly and accurately identifying patients with MTBI in an acute care setting so that proper evaluation and treatment can be rendered. Injury definitions or criteria that tend to be overinclusive could result in unnecessary utilization of resources or inaccurate diagnosis that does not identify the true underlying cause of a patient's symptoms, and therefore the inability to address those symptoms and their cause. In other words, the result is a type I error in which a condition is diagnosed where it is not actually present. A perfect demonstration of this issue is when retrospective reviews that include broad-sweeping hospital diagnostic codes such as "head injury, unspecified" categorize many patients who do not meet the clinical criteria for TBI.

A reverse phenomenon is apparent when injury definitions and criteria tend to be more restrictive or underinclusive. In this instance, the clinical risk is that true cases of MTBI will be overlooked, resulting in the failed delivery of proper evaluation and treatment. This issue is influenced by the facts that the signs and symptoms of MTBI are often poorly understood and go unrecognized, cases are sometimes missed in the context of more severe trauma (e.g., orthopedic or internal injuries) that require higher priority in critical care, and many patients do not seek any medical treatment at all after MTBI. This form of type II error is especially concerning in the case of MTBI, where reports indicate that intervention to reduce disability following MTBI is most effective when provided during the acute phase after MTBI.[23]

In a research setting, injury definitions and criteria have a significant impact on the eventual interpretation of findings on acute effects, recovery, treatment response, functional outcome, and prevalence of disability following MTBI. Specifically, some have argued that "softer" criteria that tend to be overinclusive result in a significant sampling bias that inflates the incidence of MTBI and likely overreports the occurrence of poor outcome following MTBI, some of which may well be due to non-MTBI (nonspecific) factors. As discussed in part four, sampling bias is considered to be a significant factor influencing reports on the prevalence and impact of PCS. In contrast, studies that use more restrictive criteria may tend to underreport the true incidence of MTBI and resulting disability. This, however, appears to be less of an issue than existing (hospital-based) injury surveillance systems simply not capturing cases in the first place.

4

Advances in MTBI Research Methodologies

Traditional MTBI Research Challenges

Traditional research paradigms to study MTBI have been hampered by a number of practical and methodological limitations, particularly when it comes to executing prospective studies of *acute* TBI. Until recently, there were limited data from prospective, controlled studies of *mild* TBI. Furthermore, findings from these studies are difficult to interpret based on methods that include varied injury definitions and criteria, small sample sizes with lack of adequate control groups, lack of standardized assessment of acute symptoms and cognitive functioning, limited objective follow-up assessment at varied intervals, and varied measures used to assess eventual recovery and outcome.

For instance, in the case of motor vehicle crashes, falls, assaults, or other external causes of TBI, there is often not an eye-witness account of the injury itself or the patient's acute injury characteristics (e.g., period of uncon-sciousness, PTA) to better establish MTBI-defining criteria. Inherently, there is limited reliability of information from patients who were rendered un-conscious for an undetermined period of time or are still in the throws of PTA at the point of initial critical care. Worse yet, many MTBI patients who seek no medical follow-up after their injury are never accrued into formal research studies.

Even when hospital contact is made, there is limited accessibility to injured patients to formally assess symptom severity, cognitive functioning, and other deficits with standardized measures. For instance, neuropsychological testing is quite impractical and essentially impossible to conduct in the hospital emergency department. As a result, there is often a lack of data from objective cognitive measures during the acute phase against which to track the course of recovery and eventual outcome. Finally, busy clinicians in a hospital emergency department are also typically not in a position to gather extensive premorbid history. This is especially critical given what is known about the multitude of noninjury factors that can complicate recovery after MTBI, including personality variables, mental health, alcohol and drug abuse, and personal stress.

MTBI Unknowns and Clinical Dilemmas

As a result of these challenges to traditional MTBI research, many unknowns about MTBI have persisted and left a gap for the clinician faced with evaluation and treatment of MTBI patients:

- *Diagnosis*: What is the threshold for injury? (Was there indeed an MTBI?) What are the defining characteristics of MTBI? Could there be other causes for the patient's presenting symptoms?
- *Recovery*: How long should it take to recovery after MTBI? What is the expected natural course of this injury?
- *Prognosis*: What are the acute and subacute predictors of positive and negative outcomes after MTBI?
- *Complications*: To what extent are neurologic versus psychological factors contributing to symptoms and deficits?
- *Treatment*: Given all this, what approach to treatment gives my patient the best chance for recovery?
- *Outcome*: What are the best methods to assess recovery and functional outcome after MTBI?

Innovative Approaches to MTBI Research

Researchers are always in pursuit of inventing a better mousetrap, and the evolving science of MTBI is no exception. Based on the research complications and the resulting clinical unknowns outlined above, it has become increasingly apparent that traditional paradigms used to study MTBI are insufficient to clarify the true incidence and natural history of MTBI and therefore leave gaps in the evidence base to drive clinical management of these injuries. As a result, researchers have begun to "think outside the box" in designing nontraditional, prospective studies of MTBI incidence, injury characteristics, assessment techniques, recovery—and, yes, even outcome.

Of all places, it was the sports medicine world (with help from the neurosciences) that vaulted the science of MTBI forward. Barth et al.[42] were first to recognize that many aspects inherent to sport-related concussion essentially created a laboratory for the study of MTBI. They recognized the shortcomings of earlier research, which failed to realize and methodologically control for the fact that MTBI is a different animal than more severe or complicated TBI. And, thus was born the Sports as a Laboratory Assessment Model (SLAM).[43]

The SLAM design first created by Barth and colleagues in the 1980s paved the way for other neuropsychologists and still remains the general design employed in most sport-related concussion studies to date. The fact is that the original work by Barthand colleagues still remains one of the seminal studies of sports concussion, and no studies to date have rendered findings appreciably different than those reported by Barth and colleagues more than 10 years ago. Since then, neuropsychologists have capitalized on these advantages and made a substantial contribution to the scientific literature on sport-related concussion, while also providing direct clinical services to assist in the evaluation and management of athletes following concussion. As Barth and colleagues point out, the basic science and biomechanical research communities have also now begun to capitalize on the methodological advantages of the sports concussion research model first created and since fostered by neuropsychologists.

The methodological advantages of the sports concussion research model that provide many benefits to the scientist that could not be accomplished in more traditional MTBI clinical or research contexts include the following:

UNIQUE ADVANTAGE 1: PROSPECTIVE IDENTIFICATION OF LARGE SAMPLE (ATHLETES) AT RISK OF MTBI

Access to an enormous volume of affected patients is key to accruing subjects in any area of research. Sports and recreation are among the most common causes of MTBI, particularly among teens and young adults. Recent reports suggest that sports account for more than 25 percent of MTBIs in children 5–14 years of age[23] and that approximately 5 percent of participants in organized high school and college sports experience a concussion each season.[44] In total, there are at least 300,000 reported sport-related concussions per year.[45] In high school football, for example, it is estimated that more than 40,000 concussions are reported each year; hockey, soccer, wrestling, lacrosse, and other contact sports are also known to have relative high incidence of MTBI. As is the case outside of sports, countless more injuries go unreported.[46] From the perspective of the researcher, availability of data is nearly a sure thing in the sports concussion research model.

UNIQUE ADVANTAGE 2: DEFINED PERIOD OF MTBI RISK EXPOSURE (SPORT SEASON)

In addition to the sheer volume of injuries, there is also a clear window of risk exposure (i.e., sport season) in the sports concussion research model. Across various sports with known risk of concussion, researchers can count on approximately 3–10 percent of the study sample to sustain a concussion during a three-month span of the sport season. In a football paradigm, for example, a large number of concussions can be prospectively studied each year between Labor Day and Thanksgiving, most of which will occur on Friday night. The predictability of the rate and pattern of occurrence makes it much simpler to put systems in place to accurately capture these cases and track the patient's recovery over time.

UNIQUE ADVANTAGE 3: ABILITY TO OBTAIN PREINJURY BASELINE TESTING ON THIS SAMPLE

A central tenet to the SLAM model coined by Barth and colleagues is the employment of preinjury baseline testing upon enrollment in the study for all subjects at risk of subsequent concussion.

These preinjury baseline evaluations not only include cognitive testing against which to track postinjury cognitive recovery, but also gather critical history on subjects that can be analyzed to determine how premorbid or other noninjury factors affect outcome following MTBI. The prospective nature of collecting preinjury baseline data is perhaps the key factor that distinguishes the sports concussion research model from traditional research paradigms.

UNIQUE ADVANTAGE 4: WITNESSED ACCOUNTS OF THE INJURY TO DOCUMENT ACUTE INJURY CHARACTERISTICS

As noted above, one of the challenges in most MTBI studies lies in documentation of the acute injury characteristics and essential criteria on which the case definition of MTBI is based. In hospital emergency department studies, for example, unconsciousness, amnesia, and other acute injury characteristics are frequently not documented, and collateral information sources are not available.

UNIQUE ADVANTAGE 5: ACCESSIBILITY TO CONDUCT STANDARDIZED TESTING WITHIN MINUTES OF INJURY

Contrary to traditional studies where the first data collection point is often several months postinjury, the SLAM model provides researchers with access to injured athletes on the field or sideline within minutes of MTBI. Several screening tools appropriate for the sports setting have been validated in the detection and measurement of acute symptoms, cognitive dysfunction, and postural stability resulting from MTBI. This window of accessibility truly provides us with the opportunity to capture the earliest snapshot of MTBI effects and recovery, an opportunity on which traditional MTBI research paradigms typically could not capitalize.

UNIQUE ADVANTAGE 6: SYSTEMATIC FOLLOW-UP TO TRACK EARLY RECOVERY AND OUTCOME

In addition to immediate accessibility to injured subjects, the sports concussion research model also implements a serial testing paradigm to objectively track recovery in symptoms, cognitive functioning, postural stability, and other effects of concussion during the first hours, days, and weeks postinjury. Again, the availability of individualized baseline data on these measures provides a benchmark against to track "recovery." The serial testing paradigm has afforded research a unique opportunity to refine statistical techniques to isolate clinical meaningful change in test performance from error variance and other factors that can influence the pattern of performance in both injured and non-injured subjects (e.g., practice effects upon repeated exposure). This approach has allowed researchers to, for the first time, plot the true natural history of MTBI recovery from the first several minutes to several months postinjury.

UNIQUE ADVANTAGE 7: CONTINUITY OF CARE

In a sports medicine setting, it is usually the same health care professional, most often a certified athletic trainer, who is principally responsibility for medical management of the injured athlete from diagnosis to treatment, rehabilitation, and eventual return to competition. In the case of sports concussion, this professional is often present to witness the injury event, document acute injury characteristics, administer standardized testing acutely and over the course of recovery, and determine an eventual end point to recovery. This continuity is not only beneficial from a clinical perspective but also provides a higher element of standardization and consistency to reduce the potential influence of interrater unreliability, varied documentation preferences, and other confounds common to traditional MTBI research paradigms.

UNIQUE ADVANTAGE 8: READY ACCESS TO NONINJURED CONTROLS

The team-sport nature of the sports concussion research environment provides immediate access to noninjured control subjects matched (e.g., "yoked") to each injured subject on the basis of demographics (e.g., age, gender, height, weight), educational experience (e.g., years, institution, grade point average, standardized test scores), and baseline performance on concussion assessment measures. The prevalence of orthopedic sport injuries also allows creation of an injured (non-head-injured) control group, which is now considered important for differentiating the effects of general trauma from MTBI on postconcussive symptoms and cognitive functioning. Collectively, these conditions allow researchers much tighter control than previously accomplished in MTBI research.

UNIQUE ADVANTAGE 9: RARE EVENTS

Sports are perhaps the only setting in which the MTBI patient is eager to return to the very activity that caused their injury, sometimes immediately pleading with the physician or certified athletic trainer on the sport sideline to return to competition. It is well established that many athletes indeed return to a game or practice on the same day of their injury, many while still symptomatic or impaired. Recurrent MTBI is not uncommon in sports, and the overwhelming majority of repeat concussions occur within the first several days after initial injury. This creates a unique opportunity to study the cumulative effects of multiple MTBI on immediate recovery and long-term outcome, which is essentially impossible in traditional MTBI research. The extremely rare phenomenon of so-called second impact syndrome (diffuse cerebral swelling) that is unique to sports also allows researchers to study rare occurrences of catastrophic outcome resulting from MTBI.

UNIQUE ADVANTAGE 10: "CLEAN" SAMPLE

Much has been written about the potential influence of motivational factors, litigation, and malingering on MTBI recovery. The sports concussion sample is typically free of these and other confounds encountered in traditional MTBI research. Athletes are most often highly motivated to return to competition, sometimes to the extent that they will *underreport symptoms* and *exaggerate their recovery*. Suboptimal effort on neuropsychological or other standardized testing is also extremely rare. Only recently have there been cases of sports concussion that have prompted litigation, usually alleging negligence by a health care provider that contributed to catastrophic injury or poor outcome. Theoretically, alcohol and drug abuse is also less problematic in sports concussion than in a traditional MTBI research paradigm (e.g., hospital emergency department study), at least in terms of substances on board at the time of the acute injury.

UNIQUE ADVANTAGE 11: LONGITUDINAL STUDIES

Finally, researchers have recently had success in longitudinally tracking the long-range effects. Retrospective studies have documented the potential effects of recurrent concussion during a sport career on late-life risk of depression, cognitive decline, and Alzheimer's disease.[47] The wealth of data from high school, college, and professional athletes enrolled in sports concussion studies over the past decade also provides an incredible sample that can be followed over time to prospectively study the mid-range and long-term effects of MTBI, particularly recurrent injury.

Conclusion

The goal of part one is to create perspective on the significance of MTBI and gaps in existing research that sets the table for the following discussion of scientific advances in the last decade that fill this void for the clinician. With the stated goal of this book providing the reader with a go-to shelf reference on MTBI, several summary conclusions that can be drawn from part one are summarized below.

Part One Top 10 Conclusions

1. All-severity TBI is one of the most significant public health problems in the United States and worldwide based on incidence, prevalence, health care resource utilization, resulting death and disability, and total economic cost.

2. More than 80 percent of all TBI are categorized as MTBI, with incidence rates in the order of 500/100,000 population; pinpointing the true incidence of MTBI has been hampered by a multitude of methodological factors (e.g., variable injury definitions and criteria, surveillance systems, research setting).

3. The highest rates of all-severity TBI and MTBI are observed in the very young and very old, males, minorities of low socioeconomic status, and substance abusers.

4. There is nothing "mild" about the impact of MTBI in terms of incidence, lost function, and total economic cost.

5. Traditional means for classifying TBI severity have limited utility in detecting and categorizing MTBI; multidimensional definitions that incorporate information on biomechanics, acute injury characteristics, clinical signs, symptoms, and course result in the most accurate diagnosis of MTBI.

6. Traditional MTBI research has been hampered by several methodological issues that historically have left us with many clinical unknowns about MTBI diagnosis, recovery, prognosis, treatment, and outcome.

7. New innovative approaches to MTBI research—including sports concussion studies—capitalize on several methodological advantages not previously possible in traditional MTBI research models.

8. Several prospective studies have generated groundbreaking findings over the past decade that plot the natural course of MTBI clinical effects and methodologies, provide clinicians with improved instruments for the assessment of MTBI, and establish an empirical basis to drive best clinical practice in the diagnosis and treatment of MTBI and PCS.

9. Progress has been made over the past decade in gaining a consensus definition of MTBI, implementing standardized protocols for prospective study, and applying advanced technologies position the neurosciences to address the most pressing question of all related to MTBI: What is the true natural history of MTBI?

10. The complexities of PCS are inherently linked to the science of MTBI. Scientific advances that increase our understanding of MTBI also prompt a new perspective on the definition, incidence, etiology, and diagnosis of PCS, which in turn influences the development of effective intervention models to improve outcome and reduce disability associated with MTBI and PCS.

References

1. Coronado VG, Johnson RL, Faul M, Kegler SR. Incidence rates of hospitalization related to traumatic brain injury—12 states, 2002. *MMWR Morb Mortal Wkly Rep* 2006;55(8):201–4.

2. Silver JM, McAllister TW, Yudofsky SC, eds. *Textbook of Traumatic Brain Injury*. Washington, DC: American Psychiatric Publishing, 2005.

3. Rutland-Brown W, Langlois JA, Thomas KE, Xi YL. Incidence of traumatic brain injury in the United States, 2003. *J Head Trauma Rehabil* 2006;21(6):544–8.

4. Kraus JF, Chu LD. Epidemiology. In: Silver JM, McAllister TW, Yudofsky SC, eds. *Textbook of Traumatic Brain Injury*. Washington DC: American Psychiatric Publishing, 2005; 3–26.

5. Fife D. Head injury with and without hospital admission: comparisons of incidence and short-term disability. *Am J Public Health* 1987;77:810–12.

6. Langlois JA, Rutland-Brown W, Thomas KE. The incidence of traumatic brain injury among children in the United States: differences by race. *J Head Trauma Rehabil* 2005;20(3):229–38.

7. Keenan HT, Bratton SL. Epidemiology and outcomes of pediatric traumatic brain injury. *Dev Neurosci* 2006;28(4–5):256–63.

8. Thompson HJ, McCormick WC, Kagan SH. Traumatic brain injury in older adults: epidemiology, outcomes, and future implications. *J Am Geriatr Soc* 2006;54(10):1590–95.

9. Franko J, Kish KJ, O'Connell BG, Subramanian S, Yuschak JV. Advanced age and preinjury warfarin anticoagulation increase the risk of mortality after head trauma. *J Trauma* 2006;61(1):107–10.

10. Langlois JA, Kegler SR, Butler JA, et al. Traumatic brain injury-related hospital discharges. Results from a 14-state surveillance system, 1997. *MMWR Surveill Summ* 2003;52(4):1–20.

11. Kraus JF, Fife D, Ramstein K, Conroy C, Cox P. The relationship of family income to the incidence, external causes, and outcomes of serious brain injury, San Diego County, California. *Am J Public Health* 1986;76(11):1345–47.

12. Sosin DM, Sniezek JE, Thurman DJ. Incidence of mild and moderate brain injury in the United States, 1991. *Brain Inj* 1996;10(1):47–54.

13. Langlois J, Rutland-Brown W, Wald MM. The epidemiology and impact of traumatic brain injury—a brief overview. *J Head Trauma Rehabil* 2006;21(5):375–78.

14. Coronado VG, Thomas KE, Sattin RW, Johnson RL. The CDC traumatic brain injury surveillance system: characteristics of persons aged 65 years and older hospitalized with a TBI. *J Head Trauma Rehabil* 2005;20(3): 215–28.

15. Popovic JR, Kozak LJ. National Hospital Discharge Survey: Annual Summary. National Center for Health Statistics, Centers for Disease Control and Prevention; Atlanta, GA 2000.

16. Schneier AJ, Shields BJ, Hostetler SG, Xiang H, Smith GA. Incidence of pediatric traumatic brain injury and associated hospital resource utilization in the United States. *Pediatrics* 2006;118(2):483–92.

17. Lewin ICF. *The Cost of Disorders of the Brain.* Washington, DC: National Foundation for Brain Research, 1992.

18. Langlois JA, Rutland-Brown W, Wald MM. The epidemiology and impact of traumatic brain injury: a brief overview. *J Head Trauma Rehabil* 2006;21(5):375–78.

19. Finkelstein E, Corso P, Miller T. *The Incidence and Economic Burden of Injuries in the United States.* New York: Oxford University Press, 2006.

20. *Report to Congress on Mild Traumatic Brain Injury in the United States: Steps to Prevent a Serious Public Health Problem.* Atlanta, GA: National Center for Injury Prevention and Control, Centers for Disease Control and Injury Prevention, 2003.

21. Cassidy JD, Carroll LJ, Peloso PM, et al. Incidence, risk factors and prevention of mild traumatic brain injury: results of the WHO Collaborating Centre Task Force on Mild Traumatic Brain Injury. *J Rehabil Med* 2004(43 suppl):28–60.

22. Bazarian JJ, McClung J, Shah MN, Cheng YT, Flesher W, Kraus J. Mild traumatic brain injury in the United States, 1998—2000. *Brain Inj* 2005;19(2):85–91.

23. Carroll LJ, Cassidy JD, Holm L, Kraus J, Coronado VG. Methodological issues and research recommendations for mild traumatic brain injury: the WHO Collaborating Centre Task Force on Mild Traumatic Brain Injury. *J Rehabil Med* 2004(43 suppl):113–25.

24. Bazarian JJ, Veazie P, Mookerjee S, Lerner EB. Accuracy of mild traumatic brain injury case ascertainment using ICD-9 codes. *Acad Emerg Med* 2006;13(1):31–38.

25. Max W, MacKenzie EJ, Rice DP. Head injuries: costs and consequences. *J Head Trauma Rehabil* 1991;6(2):76–91.

26. Thurman DJ. The epidemiology and economics of head trauma. In: Miller L, Hayes R, eds. *Head Trauma: Basic, Preclinical, and Clinical Directions*. New York: John Wiley and Sons, 2001.

27. Boake C, McCauley SR, Pedroza C, Levin HS, Brown SA, Brundage SI. Lost productive work time after mild to moderate traumatic brain injury with and without hospitalization. *Neurosurgery* 2005;56(5):994–1003.

28. Rimel RW, Giordani B, Barth JT, Boll TJ, Jane JA. Disability caused by minor head injury. *Neurosurgery* 1981;9(3):221–28.

29. Dikmen SS, Temkin NR, Machamer JE, Holubkov AL, Fraser RT, Winn HR. Employment following traumatic head injuries. *Arch Neurol* 1994;51(2):177–86.

30. Iverson GL, Lange RT, Gaetz M, Zasler ND. Mild TBI. In: Zafonte RD, ed. *Brain Injury Medicine: Principles and Practice*. New York: Demos Medical Publishing, 2006; 333–71.

31. Stein SC. Classification of head injury. In: Narayan RK, Povlishock JT, Wilberger JE Jr, eds. *Neurotrauma*. New York: McGraw-Hill, 1996; 31–42.

32. Jennett B, Teasdale G. *Management of Head Injuries*. Philadelphia, PA: FA Davis, 1981.

33. Davis DP, Serrano JA, Vilke GM, et al. The predictive value of field versus arrival Glasgow Coma Scale score and TRISS calculations in moderate-to-severe traumatic brain injury. *J Trauma* 2006;60(5):985–90.

34. Ommaya AK, Gennarelli TA. Cerebral concussion and traumatic unconsciousness. Correlation of experimental and clinical observations of blunt head injuries. *Brain* 1974;97(4):633–54.

35. Kay T, Harrington DE, Adams R, et al. Definition of mild traumatic brain injury. *J Head Trauma Rehabil* 1993;8(3):86–87.

36. Holm L, Cassidy JD, Carroll LJ, Borg J. Summary of the WHO Collaborating Centre for Neurotrauma Task Force on Mild Traumatic Brain Injury. *J Rehabil Med* 2005;37(3):137–41.

37. Defense and Veterans Brain Injury Center Working Group on the Acute Management of Mild Traumatic Brain Injury in Military Operational Settings: Clinical Practice Guidelines and Recommendations. Defense and Veterans Brain Injury Center. Washington, DC. December 22, 2006.

38. American Academy of Neurology. Practice parameter: the management of concussion in sports (summary statement). Report of the Quality Standards Subcommittee. *Neurology* 1997;48(3):581–85.

39. Aubry M, Cantu R, Dvorak J, et al. Summary and agreement statement of the First International Conference on Concussion in Sport, Vienna 2001. Recommendations for the improvement of safety and health of athletes who may suffer concussive injuries. *Br J Sports Med* 2002;36(1):6–10.

40. McCrory P, Johnston K, Meeuwisse W, et al. Summary and agreement statement of the 2nd International Conference on Concussion in Sport, Prague 2004. *Br J Sports Med* 2005;39(4):196–204.

41. Bazarian JJ, Blyth B, Cimpello L. Bench to bedside: evidence for brain injury after concussion—looking beyond the computed tomography scan. *Acad Emerg Med* 2006;13(2):199–214.

42. Barth JT, Freeman JR, Winters JE. Management of sports-related concussions. *Dent Clin North Am* 2000;44(1):67–83.

43. Barth JT, Freeman JR, Broshek DK, Varney RN. Acceleration-deceleration sport-related concussion: the gravity of it all. *J Athl Train* 2001;36(3):253–56.

44. Guskiewicz KM, Weaver NL, Padua DA, Garrett WE, Jr. Epidemiology of concussion in collegiate and high school football players. *Am J Sports Med* 2000;28(5):643–50.

45. Thurman DJ, Branche CM, Sniezek JE. The epidemiology of sports-related traumatic brain injuries in the United States: recent developments. *J Head Trauma Rehabil* 1998;13(2):1–8.

46. McCrea M, Hammeke T, Olsen G, Leo P, Guskiewicz K. Unreported concussion in high school football players: implications for prevention. *Clin J Sport Med* 2004;14(1):13–7.

47. Guskiewicz KM, Marshall SW, Bailes J, et al. Association between recurrent concussion and late-life cognitive impairment in retired professional football players. *Neurosurgery* 2005;57(4):719–26.

PART TWO

BASIC AND CLINICAL SCIENCE OF MTBI

While there is an extensive history of research focusing on the long-term effects of mild traumatic brain injury (MTBI) on symptoms, cognition, and daily function, the greatest advancements over the past decade relate to our understanding of the basic and clinical science of MTBI during the most acute period. Clinical studies on long-term outcome have been possible for as long as MTBI patients have been around, but technological advances have drastically catapulted forward the scientific study of the biomechanics, neurophysiology, and functional neuroanatomy that underlie the immediate clinical presentation of MTBI. Gaining perspective into the basic mechanisms of MTBI ultimately moves us closer and closer to answering the pressing question driving this text: *What is the true natural history of MTBI?* Taken further, it can be argued that addressing issues of long-term outcome is impossible without first clarifying key basic science and clinical underpinnings of any disease entity, including MTBI.

As noted in part one, there has been longstanding debate over whether persistent effects following MTBI (i.e., the basis for postconcussion syndrome [PCS]) are due to psychological *or* (not *and*) neurologic factors. In some respects, this debate has been short-sited and overly simplified as an either-or condition. That is, sometimes the very notion that MTBI can be characterized by damage to the structure and function of the brain is quickly dismissed based suspicion of psychological or non-injury-related factors as the basis for a patient's persistent or chronic complaints following MTBI.

An abundance of research over the last 10 years has now illustrated a clear neuropathophysiology of MTBI, while also clarifying the expected time course for the brain's eventual return to normal physiologic functioning after MTBI. These advances in the basic science of MTBI now put us in a much better position to interpret the persistent clinical effects of MTBI and inform our understanding of PCS.

Part two focuses on a review of findings from recent studies on the biomechanics, neurophysiology, and conventional neuroimaging of *acute* MTBI, as well as emerging evidence on the utility of functional neuroimaging techniques and biologic markers as objective indicators of brain injury. This body of work on the basic and clinical science of MTBI provides a sound empirical base on which to build our understanding of the true natural history of clinical effects and recovery after MTBI.

5

Biomechanics of MTBI

A critical component of any injury examination is reconstructing the event or accident that is considered the cause of the patient's presenting injuries. As noted in part one, this is a sometimes difficult exercise in the case of MTBI where oftentimes there are no eyewitnesses and patients are unable to provide a credible report due to a period of unconsciousness or posttraumatic amnesia that confounds their account of the incident. As a result, clinicians are often left with the challenge of determining whether or not the accident in question was sufficient to cause underlying brain injury. In a motor vehicle accident scenario, it is common to ascertain where the patient was positioned in the vehicle, whether they were belted, how fast the vehicle was traveling, the crash orientation (e.g., rear-ended vs. broadsided vs. rollover), and the nature of any direct impact to the head in the accident—all in hopes of reconstructing a biomechanical model for that individual case. In other accident scenarios, it is equally important to establish aspects of acceleration and deceleration, translational and rotational dynamics, and a general sense of injury biomechanics. Historically, establishing a *minimal biomechanical threshold* for traumatic brain injury has been one of the most elusive concepts frustrating biomechanists and neuroscience researchers.

The seminal work by Ommaya and Gennarelli[1] continues as one of the cornerstones of research on the biomechanics and neuropathology of MTBI. These researchers presented a hypothesis for cerebral concussion that outlined the principles underlying the distribution of focal and diffuse effects on neural tissues from cerebral concussion, which correlated with the clinical, experimental, and pathologic observations on blunt head trauma from that era. The Ommaya and Gennarelli definition of cerebral concussion referenced clinical, pathophysiologic, and biomechanical components as a

> graded set of clinical syndromes following head injury wherein increasing severity of disturbance in level and content of consciousness is caused by mechanically induced strains affecting the brain in a centripetal sequence of disruptive effect on function and structure. The effects of this sequence always begin at the surfaces of the brain in the mild cases and extend inwards to affect the diencephalic-mesencephalic core at the most severe levels of trauma.[1]

The Ommaya and Gennarelli system for classifying severity of concussion (i.e., MTBI) is presented in chapter 3 (see table 3.4).

The hypotheses of Ommaya and Gennarelli[1] on the biomechanics and pathophysiology of concussion led to three important predictions. First, when the level of trauma is severe enough to produce what is described as traumatic unconsciousness, the extent of simultaneous primary injury in the brain is more severe in cortical and subcortical structures than in the rostral brainstem. Second, because the mesencephalon is the last to be affected by trauma, primary damage to the rostral brainstem will not occur in isolation in the vast majority of head injuries that are associated with acceleration or deceleration trauma. Primary lesions of the rostral brainstem are rarely found post mortem, and always in association with more diffuse damage to the brain. In the case of lower grades of cerebral concussion where the patient dies from other causes, Ommaya and Gennarelli hypothesized that isolated primary rostral brainstem lesions should not be found. The third prediction from their hypothesis was that, although confusion and disturbances of memory can occur without loss of consciousness, the reverse should never be seen. Every case of head injury with a grade IV cerebral concussion according to their classification system (i.e., paralytic coma with confusion, posttraumatic amnesia, retrograde amnesia) is always associated with a period of posttraumatic amnesia, given that the mesencephalon is less vulnerable than the temporal lobes and limbic system.

Ommaya and Gennarelli went on to reiterate that these three predictions would hold only for the commonly found head injury wherein the head is accelerated or decelerated after impact. The authors cited experimental, clinical, and pathologic observations to support the validity of their hypothesis and predictions. From experimental animal models of brain injury, it was asserted that a greater number of traumatic lesions occurred in a more diffusely widespread symmetrical manner from rotational than from translational forces. In their most influential animal study, all the animals in a rotational force group exhibited neurologic evidence of experimental cerebral concussion defined as the sudden onset of paralytic coma or traumatic unconsciousness, while none of the translated force group showed this effect. This study documented the bilateral symmetry and greater severity of all lesions except intracerebral hemorrhages in the rotational force group compared to the minimally asymmetrical lesion distribution in the translational force group.[2] Clinically, injuries involving rotational forces also seem to be more significant or severe than linear impacts, in general.

Ommaya and Gennarelli also postulated, from clinical observations, that the majority of concussions do not produce paralytic coma or traumatic unconsciousness, which marked a significant departure from consensus thinking on the topic and a pivotal point in the history of our understanding of MTBI. Instead, confusion, amnesia, and any *alteration* in mental status were considered the hallmark characteristics of MTBI, which is clearly reflected in the Ommaya and Gennarelli classification system (see table 3.4). They cited the patient who was briefly "dazed" or confused but continued in a well-coordinated sensory motor activity after a sport-related concussion without subsequent recall of the episode.[2–4]

The work of Ommaya and Gennarelli also offered a reasonable explanation for the greater vulnerability of memory and lesser vulnerability of alertness after concussion, which today serves as the basis for the cholinergic hypothesis that is discussed further below along with other supporting data on the pathophysiology of MTBI.

Most important, the early work by Ommaya and Gennarelli underscored the importance of animal models and the later development of mathematical and physical models as the *in vivo* laboratory for the study of brain injury biomechanics. There has since been a steady progression in the development of experimental models on traumatic brain injury, including paradigms that illustrate the underlying biomechanical principles of MTBI.

More recently, this movement has progressed closer and closer toward answering the elusive unknown of establishing a minimal biomechanical threshold for MTBI. Recent studies[5] have compared various MTBI experimental models and made recommendations regarding specific weight-height-impact parameters that are most appropriate and simplest for simulating the biomechanics of MTBI. This critical evaluation of various experimental models concludes that some models result in effects more reflective of severe head injury, while specific parameters show effects more consistent with MTBI.

Over the past decade, several studies have used a combination of video analysis and dummy reenactments of impacts from a sports setting as methods of head acceleration measurement. These studies[6-9] investigated concussive impacts that were recorded on film from two or more different angles. They used this videotape to reconstruct the angle of the impact, speed of the impact, and resultant player kinematics, which provided the necessary information to recreate the impact conditions with instrumented Hybrid III crash dummies in the biomechanical laboratory.

Pellman and colleagues have published a series of reports on concussion in professional football, including data on the location and direction of helmet impacts.[8-10] In a 2003 report,[8] 31 impacts were constructed with the helmeted Hybrid III dummies involving 25 concussions. This study was the first to illustrate the location, direction, and severity of helmet impacts causing concussion in National Football League players, as defined by analysis from game video and laboratory reconstruction. From these reconstructions, concussion occurred with the lowest peak head acceleration in facemask impacts at 78g ($\pm$ 18g) versus an average of 107–117g for impacts on other quadrants of the head. There was also a significantly higher head acceleration for concussed versus nonconcussed players.

In 2004, Zhang et al.[11] attempted to delineate injury causation and establish a meaningful injury criterion through the use of actual field accident data from mild traumatic brain injuries in American football, providing what the authors referred to as a unique living "laboratory" to study concussion biomechanics and tolerance levels in humans, with possible extrapolation to the general population. Again, accident reconstruction using an anatomically detailed model facilitated the prediction of the extent and severity of brain response as a consequence of a particular impact.

Zhang and colleagues assert that their approach was unlike previous studies that proposed tolerance limits for human head injury based on input kinematics scaled from either animal data or noninjurious volunteer test results. A total of 24 head-to-head field collisions that occurred in professional football games were duplicated, using a validated finite element human head model. Injury predictors and injury levels were analyzed based on resulting brain tissue responses and were correlated with the site and occurrence of MTBI. Predictions indicated that the sheer stress around the brainstem region could be an injury predictor for concussion, and statistical analyses were performed to establish a new brain injury tolerance level. Specifically, based on linear logistic regression analyses, the predicted sheer stress response in the upper brainstem was the best injury predictor over the other brain response parameters. A sheer stress of 7.8 kPa was proposed as the tolerance level for a 50 percent probability of sustaining an MTBI. Contrary to earlier studies, their analyses indicated that the translational head acceleration had a greater influence on intracranial pressure response in comparison with rotational acceleration, and the sheer stress in the central part of the brain was more sensitive to rotational acceleration than to translational acceleration.

Zhang et al.[11] concluded that if the head was exposed to a combined translational and rotational acceleration, with an impact duration of between 10 and 30 msec, the suggested tolerable reversible brain injury level was less than 85g for translational acceleration. The maximum resultant translational acceleration at the center of gravity was estimated to be 66g, 82g, and 106g for a 25 percent, 50 percent, and 80 percent probability of MTBI, respectively. For rotational acceleration, the suggested tolerable reversible brain injury level was less than 6.0×10^3 rad/sec^2. The maximum resultant rotational accelerations for a 25 percent, 50 percent, and 80 percent probability of sustaining an MTBI were estimated to be 4.6×10^3, 5.9×10^3, and 7.9×10^3 rad/sec^2, respectively.

Other researchers[12] have argued that dependence on video reconstruction and dummy reenactments creates an indirect measure of head acceleration that is limited by dummy biofidelity assumptions and validation from 30 Hz video. In addition, previous research has not given real-time information on the direction and magnitude of the impacts that football players receive. Therefore, there has been a critical need for real-time measurement of head accelerations that can be readily applied to a larger number of individuals at risk of TBI exposure (e.g., athletes participating in collision sports). Recognizing the limitations of video reconstruction and dummy reenactments, more recent technologies have focused on an innovative in-helmet system that measures and records linear head acceleration.

Brolinson et al.[12] conducted a study using the Head Impact Telemetry (HIT) system, an in-helmet system with six spring-mounted accelerometers and an antenna that transmits data via radio frequency to a sideline receiver and laptop computer system. A total of 11,604 head impacts were recorded from a college football team throughout the 2003 and 2004 football seasons during 22 games and 62 practices from a total of 52 players. The incidence of injury data was limited, but the study presented an extremely large data set from human head impacts that provides valuable insight into the lower limits of head acceleration that cause MTBI.

The average linear acceleration in the Brolinson et al. study was 20.1g ($\pm$18.7g) in the 11,601 impacts that did not result in concussion,[12] which was considerably lower than the average for noninjured players of 60g ($\pm$24g) previously reported by Pellman et al.[9] The Brolinson et al. study, however, included all head impacts during practices and games, compared with the selection of more severe open field impacts reported by Pellman et al.[9] The Brolinson et al. data are more similar to the 29.2g average head impact acceleration measured by Naunheim et al.[13] for high school players that included all impacts, not just the most severe. The three brain injuries that occurred in instrumented players in the Brolinson et al. study had a peak linear head acceleration of 55.7g, 136.7g, and 117.6g, for an average peak linear head acceleration of 103.3g.

Guskiewicz and colleagues extended the work of Brolinson et al., using the HIT system in the study of concussive and nonconcussive impacts in collegiate football players.[14–18] As part of an ongoing study, more than 27,000 impacts were recorded and analyzed for all exposures in games and practice during a single season. This study also allowed analysis of impact frequency and magnitude, while correlating biomechanical instrumentation data with clinical assessment measures following concussion. In total, nine concussions were observed in HIT-equipped players. The average magnitude of concussion impacts was 95g, with a range of 60–120g. Six of the nine concussive events had peak accelerations in excess of 95g. This compares to less than 1 percent of the 27,000 nonconcussive impacts that had a peak head acceleration in excess of 95g. It also should be pointed out, however, that even the overwhelming majority of impacts greater than 80g did not result in concussion, suggesting that a minimum threshold of translational force in this range is necessary but not solely sufficient to cause MTBI.[19]

Conclusion

In summary, several studies using video reconstruction, technologically advanced crash dummies, or even live instrumentation of human sport participants now provide us with data that start to establish a minimal threshold of peak head acceleration that provides valuable insight into the lower limits of head acceleration that cause MTBI. Across studies, there is suggestion of a minimum threshold for linear gravitational acceleration in the range of 80–100g.

The influence of rotational forces, however, must be considered in this equation as a mediating factor that may lower the necessary threshold of a translational force that causes MTBI. As suggested years ago by Ommaya and Gennarelli,[1] the addition of rotational forces greatly increases the likelihood of MTBI. Duration and location of impact can also modify the relative influence of translational force. In essence, the proposed minimum threshold for linear gravitational acceleration appears to be necessary, but not solely sufficient, to cause MTBI, as impacts of this magnitude can be observed without the occurrence of brain injury.

In real-world terms, it has been suggested that a 100g translational force is equivalent to a 25 mile-per-hour motor vehicle collision into a brick wall, striking one's head against the dash.[19] Instrumentation advancements now provide a first-ever laboratory opportunity to study the biomechanics of MTBI *in vivo* and allow us to correlate biomechanical data with clinical measures of effects and recovery associated with MTBI. In a clinical setting, these data suggesting a minimal biomechanical threshold for the occurrence of MTBI should be considered when determining if the accident in question was sufficient to cause brain injury and whether the biomechanics correlate with the severity of the patient's clinical presentation.

6

■ ■ ■

Neurophysiology of MTBI:
The Neurometabolic Cascade

The physiology of concussion (i.e., MTBI) has been nicely delineated by several scientific breakthroughs in the past decade, work that has been summarized in great detail as part of several recent reviews.[20,21] In brief, scientific advances have overhauled theories of the pathophysiology underlying all forms of neuronal injury, including MTBI. Historically, it was often assumed that the clinical manifestation of signs and symptoms following MTBI was due to destruction or sheering of neuronal axons. Therein lies the confusion that the underlying neurophysiology of MTBI is exclusively "diffuse axonal injury" (DAI). An extensive body of work over the past three decades, however, demonstrates that most of the pathophysiology of MTBI renders neurons *dysfunctional*, but not destroyed.[22]

Iverson and colleagues[22,23] have provided excellent reviews of the neuropathology of MTBI. They specifically cite the ground-breaking work of Giza and Hovda, which is eloquently summarized in a 2001 report on the pathophysiology of concussion.[24] As Iverson et al.[23] point out,

> It was once considered that excessive acceleration/deceleration forces caused sheer strains on the brain that resulted in tearing or stretching of neurons at the time of the injury. Further, it was considered that brainstem was the focus of injury. Taken together, these studies have led numerous clinicians and researchers to conclude that acceleration/deceleration injuries result in sheer strains within the cranial vault, and these in turn lead to

sheering of neurons and blood vessels occurring principally in the brainstem. Although no one doubts the existence of sheering strains as the primary pathophysiological mechanism responsible for damage to axons, the pathophysiology sequence that leads to traumatic injury of the neurons is a "process, not an event."[23,25]

Based on an extensive review of the literature, Iverson and others have pointed out that cell death following MTBI, which is considered extremely rare, reflects a spectrum of necrosis, on a continuum between apoptotic and necrotic mechanisms.[23,26] These researchers also assert that cell death is closely related to injury severity: very mild concussions likely produce virtually no permanent damage to cells resulting in long-term symptoms or problems, whereas severe traumatic brain injuries, especially those involving considerable forces, often produce widespread cellular death and dysfunction with clear functional consequences.

Recent research demonstrates that cellular injury does not specifically involve brainstem structures, contrary to previous theories. As Iverson et al.[23] point out, the continuum of injury, at the cellular level, ranges from complete and rapidly reversible cellular dysfunction (in the mildest form of MTBI), to slow but complete recovery (moderate TBI), to slow and incomplete recovery, to cell death (severe TBI). At the former end of the continuum, the pattern of complete and rapid reversal of neuronal dysfunction correlates very closely with the natural clinical history of MTBI, as discussed further in part three.

In terms of its pathophysiology, concussion (i.e., MTBI) is defined as any transient neurologic dysfunction resulting from a biomechanical force.[24] The clinical manifestation of MTBI results from sequential neuronal dysfunction due to ionic shifts, altered metabolism, impaired connectivity, or changes in neurotransmission. Collectively, the underlying pathophysiologic processes of MTBI have been characterized as a "neurometabolic cascade."[24] The stepwise stages of this process as proposed by Giza and Hovda[24] are summarized in Box 6.1 and illustrated in Figure 6.1.

The Neurometabolic Cascade

Upon impact with sufficient biomechanical force to cause MTBI (presumably with a minimum threshold of 80–100g translational acceleration), a process of abrupt and indiscriminant release of neurotransmitters and ionic flux ensues. Excitatory transmitters, including glutamate, bind to the N-methyl-D-aspartate (NMDA) receptor, leading to further neuronal depolarization and efflux of potassium and influx of calcium to affected cells. This process of ionic shift leads to acute and subacute changes in the overall cellular physiology of the brain.[24]

During the acute phase, the sodium-potassium pump works exceedingly in an attempt to restore the neuronal membrane to its normal potential. As a result, the sodium-potassium pump requires increasing amounts of adenosine triphosphate (ATP), which triggers a dramatic jump in glucose metabolism. In animal studies, increases in glucose metabolism occur almost immediately after fluid percussion injury and persist for up to 30 min in the

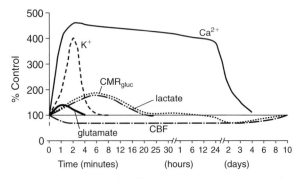

FIGURE 6.1. Neurometabolic cascade following experimental concussion (MTBI). K^+, potassium; Ca^{2+}, calcium; CMR_{gluc}, oxidative glucose metabolism; CBF, cerebral blood flow. Reprinted from Giza and Hovda,[24] with permission.

ipsilateral cortex and hippocampus.[27] The period of increased glucose metabolism is extended perhaps up to several hours and into distant areas of the brain following more severe injury, such as cortical contusion (i.e., "complicated MTBI").

This state of hypermetabolism occurs in a state of diminished cerebral blood flow, with the disparity between glucose supply and demand triggering a generalized cellular energy crisis. Cerebral blood flow is normally tightly coupled to neuronal activity and cerebral glucose metabolism, but may be reduced by 50 percent in animal fluid percussion models. In a setting of hyperglycolysis, this mismatch in supply and demand results in a potentially damaging energy crisis. This energy crisis is thought to be the likely mechanism for postconcussive vulnerability, making the brain less able to respond adequately to a second injury and potentially leading to longer lasting deficits.[24]

Beyond the initial accelerated glucose utilization, the concussed brain goes into a period of depressed metabolism. Elevated calcium levels persist and can impair mitochondrial oxidative metabolism and amplify the energy crisis. In experimental animal concussion models, the accumulation of calcium is evident within hours and may persist for up to two to four days.[28–31] Persistent and dysregulated calcium accumulation can also contribute to cell death. Intraaxonal calcium flux can disrupt neurofilaments and microtubules that ultimately impair posttraumatic neural connectivity.[24]

The significant influx of calcium can result in mitochondrial calcium accumulation and impaired oxidative metabolism, ultimately resulting in energy failure. In animal studies, oxidative metabolism shows a biphasic reduction;

in the ipsilateral cortex, a relative reduction on day 1 recovers by day 2, then reoccurs on day 3, and bottoms out on day 5, with recovery by 10 days post-injury. Smaller but more lasting changes have been recorded in the ipsilateral hippocampus, with decreases in oxidative metabolism evident for up to 10 days postinjury.[32]

Cerebral oxidative metabolism normally runs near its maximum in a steady state, so abrupt increase in energy requirements necessitates an increase in glycolysis, or *hyperglycolisis*. Mitochondrial dysfunction associated with impaired oxidative metabolism can lead to reduced ATP production, which provides a second stimulus for increased glycolysis. Increased lactate production in conjunction with decreased lactate metabolism ultimately results in lactate accumulation that can result in neuronal dysfunction by inducing acidosis, membrane damage, altered blood–brain barrier permeability, and cerebral edema.[33–37]

Following the initial phase of hyperglycolysis, cerebral glucose use is diminished by 24 hr postinjury in animal models and remains below normal levels for five to seven days in experimental animals.[27] Positron emission tomography (PET) studies in humans show similar decreases in global cerebral glucose metabolism that may last two to four weeks post-TBI[38] in more severe forms of TBI,[38] but it is unclear how these effects might present in concussion or milder forms of TBI.

Intracellular magnesium levels are immediately reduced after TBI and remain low for up to four days.[39–42] A decrease in magnesium levels may lead to neuronal dysfunction by multiple pathways; both glycolytic and oxidative generation of ATP is impaired when magnesium levels are low. Also, magnesium is necessary for maintaining the cellular membrane potential and initiating protein synthesis. Finally, low magnesium levels may effectively unblock the NMDA receptor channel more easily, leading to greater influx of calcium and its potential deleterious intracellular consequences.

Giza and Hovda[24] assert that long-term deficits in memory and cognition following all-severity MTBI may result from dysfunctional excitatory neurotransmission, including alterations in glutamatergic (NMDA), adrenergic, and cholinergic systems. Specifically, long-term potentiation, an NMDA-dependent measure of neuronal plasticity, may be persistently impaired in the hippocampus after MTBI.[43–45] MTBI may also lead to early changes in choline acetyltransferase activity and degeneration of cholinergic neurons.[46,47] The biomechanical threshold or magnitude of injury required to trigger this cascade and the specific application to MTBI in humans are not entirely clear.

Theoretically, impaired cholinergic neurotransmission leads to impairments in new learning and memory, as evidenced in other conditions separate from MTBI (e.g., Alzheimer's disease). The cholinergic theory has asserted that cholinergic neurons are particularly abundant in the hippocampus and nucleus basalis of Meynert, and are preferentially affected in animal percussion models of MTBI. Acutely, disruption of the cholinergic system is characterized clinically by a disruption in level of alertness (consciousness), which is not due to a disruption of the reticular activating system per se. Clinically, this disruption of the cholinergic system manifests as posttraumatic amnesia or anterograde memory impairment, now considered the cognitive functions most sensitive to the clinical effects of concussion, which are discussed in greater detail in part three.

Serum Biochemical Markers of MTBI

Along with advances in our understanding of the pathophysiology underlying MTBI, there is also pursuit toward identifying biochemical markers that may result in a more sensitive and objective detection of MTBI. Several studies have investigated the diagnostic and prognostic value of various biochemical markers, the most common of which are S-100 proteins, neuron-specific enolase (NSE), and cleaved tau protein (CTP). The most extensive body of research has focused on the S-100B neuroprotein, which is considered a generally reliable marker for brain damage.[48–55]

S-100B is a calcium-binding protein that is found in high concentrations in astroglial and Schwann cells, most heavily distributed in the central nervous system. It is hypothesized that S-100B is rapidly released into cerebrospinal fluid (CSF), then crosses the blood–CSF barrier upon cell damage. Several studies have reported higher concentrations of S-100B in MTBI patients than in noninjured controls.[51,54,56,57] S-100B levels are also reported to correlate with the structural abnormalities on brain neuroimaging.[23]

Several individual studies have rendered informative findings on the utility of S-100B as a marker for MTBI. Bazarian et al.[58] studied the relationship of serum S-100B and CTP levels to long-term outcome after MTBI. A total of 35 MTBI subjects presenting to the hospital emergency department were studied, with 6-hour serum S-100B and CTP levels compared to three-month outcome on PCS questionnaires. A weak correlation was demonstrated between marker levels and scores on the Rivermead postconcussion questionnaire (S-100B, $R = 0.071$; CTP, $R = 0.21$), and there was no statistically significant correlation between acute marker levels and three-month PCS. Overall, the sensitivity of these two biochemical markers ranged from 43.8 to 56.3 percent, and the specificity ranged from 35.7 to 71.4 percent. Bazarian et al. concluded that initial serum S-100B and CTP levels appear to be poor predictors of three-month outcome after MTBI.

Another concern about the S-100B biochemical marker is its extracranial release, because elevated S-100B levels have been found in non-head-injured patients and healthy sport participants. Bazarian et al.[58] later studied the impact of a correction factor for extracranial release of S-100B based on concomitant creatine kinase (CK) levels. Both CK and S-100B levels were measured in a cohort of 96 MTBI patients, which yielded a comparison of corrected S-100B and uncorrected S-100B levels for the prediction of initial head computed tomography (CT) results, three-month headache, and three-month PCS. Corrected S-100B levels resulted in a statistically significant improvement in the prediction of three-month headache, but not PCS or initial head CT. Applying a cutoff score that maximized sensitivity improved corrected S-100B's prediction of initial head CT. The researchers concluded that S-100B is poorly predictive of outcome, but that a correction factor using CK may be a valid means of accounting for extracranial release. They also proposed that by increasing the portion of MTBI patients correctly categorized as low-risk for abnormal CT, CK-corrected S-100B can further correct the number of unnecessary brain CT scans performed after MTBI.

Begaz et al.[59] recently published a collective review of prospective cohort studies that assess the ability of serum biochemical markers to predict MTBI and PCS. A total of 11 studies assessing S-100B protein, NSE, and CTP were reviewed. The authors concluded that none of these biomarkers consistently demonstrated the ability to predict PCS after MTBI, but that a combination of clinical factors in conjunction with biochemical markers may be necessary to develop a comprehensive decision rule that more accurately predicts PCS after MTBI.

Iverson et al.[23] also provided a detailed summary of sensitivity, specificity, and predictive power values of S-100B levels to predict outcome following MTBI. A series of studies between 1999 and 2004 was reviewed, with sensitivity values ranging from 80 to 100 percent, and specificity values ranging from 40.5 to 81 percent. Positive predictive power values ranged from 13 to 40.5, with negative predictive power values between 95.1 and 100. Iverson et al. concluded that the existing body of research suggests that although S-100B is not useful for identifying individuals who are "at risk" of poor outcome from TBI (i.e., positive predictive power), it is useful for identifying those individuals who are "not at risk" of poor outcome from TBI (i.e., negative predictive power; individuals who will have good outcome postinjury).

As a diagnostic tool, the practical implication of this finding from Iverson et al.'s review of the literature is that S-100B measures will misidentify a significant portion of individuals "not at risk" (i.e., expected good outcome) as being "at risk," (i.e., potential risk for poor outcome). That is, the test will be positive and they will falsely be labeled as being at risk for poor outcome. Theoretically, this could lead to unnecessary treatment or unnecessary worry for the patient.

Conclusion

In summary, basic science advances have clarified the components and sequence of the pathophysiology underlying the clinical presentation of MTBI. Existing evidence suggests a period of metabolic dysfunction that ensues after MTBI, with rapid reversal and return to normal brain metabolic function within several days of injury in most cases of concussion, and perhaps extended a bit further in more severe or "complicated" forms of MTBI characterized by structural damage visualized on neuroimaging.

This time course is strikingly similar to that illustrated by emerging data plotting the true natural history of the clinical effects of MTBI on symptoms, cognition, and general function, as discussed further in part three. Modern technologies also now open the door for the future development of innovative laboratory tests that may provide more objective markers of traumatic brain injury, perhaps with a threshold sufficient for detection of MTBI. Further study is required to determine the incremental diagnostic and prognostic utility of biologic markers of MTBI.

7

■ ■ ■

Neuroimaging in MTBI

Perhaps the most elusive exercise in the science of MTBI has been the continual pursuit of "objective" findings to demonstrate either underlying structural or functional abnormalities as markers of traumatic injury. The emergency management of MTBI typically centers on the decision to perform a head CT scan because of its utility in detecting hemorrhagic lesions and other structural injury that may require neurosurgical intervention or more acute triage. Therein lies the dilemma: while CT scans have great value in detecting neurosurgical emergencies, they also have the poorest sensitivity in detecting underlying abnormalities associated with milder forms of brain injury, including MTBI. The absence of focal findings on a CT scan is often incorrectly and inappropriately equated with a complete lack or nonexistence of brain injury, which then creates confusion among health care providers that often follows patients throughout their clinical management after injury. There is a continual pursuit in the neurosciences to develop imaging techniques sensitive to detecting structural and functional abnormalities following milder forms of brain injury, even in the absence of traumatic abnormalities on head CT scan.

The distinction between normal and abnormal imaging after MTBI can have important diagnostic and prognostic implications. Diagnostically, when clinical neuroimaging reveals abnormalities after MTBI, the classification changes to "complicated MTBI," as opposed to "uncomplicated MTBI" in which imaging studies are negative. Prognostically, injury sufficient to cause structural damage visualized on neuroimaging often results in outcome more consistent with moderate TBI.[60] The critical diagnostic and prognostic distinctions between complicated and uncomplicated are discussed further in part three.

The potential utility of more sensitive imaging techniques is especially intriguing in cases where a patient remains symptomatic despite negative conventional imaging (e.g., CT, magnetic resonance imaging [MRI]). Because the majority of MTBI patients have normal structural MRI and CT scans, there is increasing attention directed at finding objective physiologic correlates of persistent cognitive and neuropsychiatric symptoms through experimental neuroimaging techniques.[61] In recent years, an increasing number of studies have applied advanced MRI techniques, functional MRI (fMRI), PET, single-photon-emission computed tomography (SPECT) scanning, and other imaging modalities in the study of MTBI, work that is summarized in an excellent review of the literature by Belanger et al.[61] Part four presents a review of findings from recent studies that specifically applied these various imaging techniques in the study of MTBI.

Computed Tomography (CT)

With increasing pressures on hospital emergency and critical care departments to provide efficient triage and intelligent resource utilization, the CT scan is the most common and often the only radiologic technique used to evaluate traumatic brain injury. According to the National Center for Health Statistics,[62] more than 576,000 Americans undergo a head CT in hospital emergency departments for the evaluation of MTBI every year. An estimated 3–10 percent of these CT scans reveal a traumatic abnormality, and less than 1 percent require neurosurgical intervention.[63]

Iverson et al.,[64] however, reported that 15.8 percent of 912 patients with MTBI had abnormalities on their day of injury CT scan. Additionally, nearly 25 percent of the sample did not undergo CT scanning at all, mostly because their injuries were very mild, with Glasgow Coma Scale (GCS) scores of 15. Previous studies have reported similar results in the order of 10–15 percent in MTBI patients that were scanned, without taking into consideration those subjects that had no imaging conducted at all.[65–67] Based on this combination, Iverson et al. concluded that the actual prevalence of traumatic abnormalities on CT scanning in MTBI is more likely in the range of 16–21 percent.

The most common abnormalities on CT after concussion include cerebral contusions, subdural hematomas, epidural hematomas, and edema. One qualification here, as pointed out by Bazarian et al.,[58] is that CT scans detect blood and edema, but do not directly detect neuronal injury itself. It is assumed that if there is damage to more durable blood vessels, then adjacent neurons that are more vulnerable to trauma are also damaged enough to cause neuronal dysfunction (not necessarily *death*).

Researchers have also pointed out significant overlap in the acute injury characteristics for patients with ("complicated MTBI") and without ("uncomplicated MTBI") abnormalities on CT scan after MTBI.[64] Iverson et al.[64] reported that many patients with CT abnormalities had a maximum score of 15 on the GCS, sustained no loss of consciousness, and had normal performance on the Galveston Orientation and Amnesia Test (GOAT) during the acute injury phase. On a group basis, however, MTBI patients with positive findings on CT had lower GCS scores, greater frequency of loss of consciousness, higher incidence of skull fracture, and lower GOAT scores.[64]

In 2006, Iverson et al.[68] studied a cohort of 100 MTBI patients who underwent day-of-injury CT scans and then completed a small battery of neuropsychological tests within two weeks of injury. The larger group was divided into 50 subjects with normal ("uncomplicated MTBI") and 50 subjects with abnormal CT scans ("complicated MTBI"). The study demonstrated that patients with complicated MTBI's performed significantly more poorly on select neuropsychological measures, but the effect sizes were small or medium, and the two groups could not be differentiated in their eventual clinical outcome using logistic regression analysis.

Iverson et al. concluded that structural brain damage visualized on CT scanning increases the risk for slow or incomplete recovery but does not provide a perfectly predictable explanation for good or poor outcome in the majority of patients. This summation remains the most accurate depiction of the current literature on diagnostic and prognostic value of CT scanning in MTBI.

Magnetic Resonance Imaging (MRI)

Although not used as commonly in hospital emergency departments and critical care units, MRI is showing promise as a more sensitive neuroimaging method than CT for detecting subtle structural abnormalities following MTBI. There are several advantages to MRI, both methodologically and clinically, including enhanced sensitivity for detecting small intracranial abnormalities and axonal injury.[69]

When looking at all levels of TBI severity, MRI is more sensitive in detecting structural traumatic abnormalities than CT. MRI is said to be up to 25–30 percent more sensitive than CT scanning in revealing DAI,[70] but both CT and MRI are typically normal and have very weak correlation with clinical outcome after MTBI.[71] Cortical contusions, subdural hematomas, and hemorrhagic changes in the white matter are the most common findings on brain MRI after MTBI.

Bazarian[58] eloquently summarizes the results of four studies focused on MRI application following MTBI,[72–75] Those four studies reported the prevalence of MRI abnormalities after MTBI in the range of 10–57 percent, including 30 percent who had abnormalities on brain MRI but normal CT.

Hughes et al.[75] studied a series of 80 MTBI patients using MRI and neuropsychological testing during the acute phase, followed by a PCS assessment and return to work status update at six months postinjury. Twenty-six of the 80 subjects (33 percent) had abnormalities on MRI, of which only "five were definitely traumatic." The investigators report a weak correlation between MRI abnormalities and functional impairments on neuropsychological testing during the acute period, but there was no significant correlation between MRI abnormalities and eventual PCS or return to work status.

Kurca et al.[76] studied 30 MTBI patients and 30 age- and sex-matched controls with brain MRI and neuropsychological testing within 96 hr after injury. Nine of the 30 MTBI subjects had pathologic findings (traumatic or nonspecific) on brain MRI, including seven of the nine (so, 7 out of 30, 23 percent) with traumatic lesions. Nonspecific white matter lesions were found in five healthy controls (out of 30, so base nontraumatic abnormality rate of 17 percent). Investigators reported statistically significant neuropsychological difference between the MTBI patients with true traumatic lesions (complicated MTBI) and those with nonspecific lesions or normal brain MRI (uncomplicated MTBI) during the acute stage within four days of injury. The study did not include any longer term follow-up of patients to determine the prognostic value of acute MRI findings in predicting functional outcome.

In general, MRI techniques are more sensitive than CT in detecting subtle, specific abnormalities after MTBI, but have limited utility in identifying or predicting delayed recovery or persistent problems after MTBI, much like CT.[23]

Diffusion Tensor Imaging (DTI)

Recent studies have investigated the utility of diffusion tensor MRI in traumatic brain injury, particularly in an attempt to detect and characterize underlying DAI. DTI is a relatively new MRI application that capitalizes on the diffusion of water molecules for imaging the brain. While diffusion-weighted

MRI measures the diffusion of water molecules in a particular direction, DTI extends this technology by imaging diffusion in several different directions (e.g., six).[61]

DTI is especially sensitive to measuring integrity of white matter tracts and critical structures. Fractional anisotropy (FA) is the most robust DTI metric and provides a measure of tissue microstructure by quantifying the extent to which diffusion occurs in one particular direction within each voxel.[61] Preliminary data[77] suggested that DTI is sensitive to detecting reduced FA in white matter (most prominent in the internal capsule and corpus callosum) during the acute and subacute period postinjury in MTBI cases who had normal-appearing white matter on conventional MRI. The same study indicated recovery in white matter abnormalities on DTI one month postinjury.

Inglese et al.[78] studied 46 MTBI patients (loss of consciousness < 20 min, posttraumatic amnesia < 24 hr, GCS score of 13–15) and 20 healthy volunteer controls who underwent MRI with dual-spin echo, fluid-attenuated inversion recovery, T_2-weighted gradient echo, and DTI sequences. Twenty MTBI patients underwent imaging an average of 4.05 days after injury, and the other 26 subjects were imaged an average of 5.7 years after MTBI. In each case, mean diffusivity and fractional anisotropy were measured using both whole-brain histograms in regions of interest (ROI) analyses. No differences in any of the histogram-derived measures were found between patients and control volunteers. Compared with controls, a significant reduction of fractional anisotropy was observed in patient's corpus callosum, internal capsule, and centrum semiovale, and there were significant increases of mean diffusivity in the corpus callosum and internal capsule. Neither histogram-derived nor regional DTI metrics differed between the two (acute vs. chronic MTBI) groups.

The investigators concluded that although mean diffusivity and fractional anisotropy abnormalities in patients with MTBI are too subtle to be detected with whole-brain histogram analysis, they were present in brain areas known to be preferentially effected by DAI. Finally, they concluded that because DTI changes are present at both early and late times following injury, they may represent an early indicator and prognostic measure of subsequent brain damage.

Belanger et al.[61] summarize the literature by suggesting that DTI may be in a unique position to predict recovery in TBI patients, with particular relevance to MTBI that results in axonal injury (not death) not identified on normal CT/MRI scans.

Magnetic Transfer Imaging (MTI) and Magnetic Source Imaging (MSI)

Magnetic transfer imaging (MTI) is a technique that exploits the exchange of protons between water and macromolecules to increase the visualized contrast between tissues, which is not detected on conventional T_1- and T_2-weighted MRI. A magnetization ratio (MTR) provides a quantitative measure of tissue structural integrity, with a reduced MTR suggestive of neuronal dysfunction or neuropathology. Preliminary studies suggest that MTI is sensitive to detection of abnormalities not captured by traditional MRI, although these studies have included a mixture of all-severity TBI, and correlation with clinical outcome has been weak.[61,79]

Belanger et al.[61] summarize the literature by stating that MTI with MTBI patients largely detects abnormalities within the first one to two months after injury, and that demonstrated areas of abnormality on MTI are general consistent with the known neuropathology of MTBI (i.e., regional abnormalities in lobar white matter and corpus callosum), but further study is required to determine the diagnostic and prognostic value of these findings.

MSI acquires electrophysiologic data from the brain through the use of magnetoencephalography and combines it with data on structural brain integrity from conventional MRI. Limited data is available on MSI in MTBI, suggesting that MSI appears to be sensitive in cases of MTBI with persistent postconcussive complaints (up to three times more sensitive than conventional MRI alone), but not necessarily in all MTBI patients,[61,80] which leaves questions about the clinical sensitivity and specificity of MSI in MTBI. The clinical significance of MSI has also not been correlated with functional outcome.

Magnetic Resonance Spectroscopy (MRS)

A limited number of recent, small studies have investigated the utility of MRS and MTBI. Govindaraju et al.[81] studied 14 subjects with MTBI who underwent structural MRI and proton MRS within one month of injury. The results were compared with data from 13 noninjured controls. Investigators reported significant changes in some, but not all, brain regions for the average values of all MTBI subjects, with reduced N-acetyl aspartate (NAA), total creatinine (CR), increased total choline (CHO)/CR, and reduced NAA/CHO. These metabolic ratios were calculated for 25 regions without MRI abnormalities. Metabolic ratios were not significantly correlated with GCS score at admission or Glasgow Outcome Scale score at six months after injury.

The investigators assert that these results showed evidence of widespread metabolic changes following MTBI in regions that appeared normal on diagnostic MRI. Although any association with injury assessment and outcome was weak, these findings raise question as to the possible utility of volumetric proton MRS for evaluating diffuse injury following MTBI. Other studies using studies of MRS in MTBI are confounded by the inclusion of more severe TBI patients, concurrent abnormalities on structural imaging either on CT or MRI, or the lack of any correlation with functional outcome.

Functional Magnetic Resonance Imaging (fMRI)

Emerging technologies in neuroimaging are designed to detect abnormalities in brain function, not just structural integrity, which provide promise given theories of neuronal dysfunction following MTBI, in the absence of structural lesions per se. fMRI has better temporal and spatial resolution than other functional imaging modalities and, consequently, when combined with structural MRI, provides more accurate mapping of the brain structure to function than PET or SPECT.[82]

Over the past five years, several studies have applied fMRI in the investigation of TBI, including investigations of mild TBI. The work of McAllister and colleagues has been at the forefront of this movement. Several studies by this research group have studied the effects of MTBI on working memory through the use of fMRI techniques. In a 1999 study, McAllister et al.[83] reported different brain activation patterns between MTBI patients and control subjects on fMRI in response to increasing working memory processing loads using an N-back cognitive paradigm. In this particular study, 12 MTBI patients were studied with fMRI within one month of injury and compared to 11 healthy control subjects.

Control subjects showed bifrontal and biparietal activation in response to a low processing load, with a minimal increase in activation associated with the high-load task. MTBI patients, however, showed some activation during the low-processing-load task but significantly increased activation during the high-load condition, particularly in the right parietal and right dorsolateral frontal regions. The investigators initially concluded that MTBI patients differed from control subjects in activation patterns of working memory circuitry in response to different processing loads, despite similar task performance, which suggested that injury-related changes in ability to activate or to modulate working memory processing resources may underlie some of the memory complaints after MTBI.

A subsequent published report by McAllister et al. in 2001[82] again showed differential working memory load effects after MTBI, where MTBI patients showed disproportionately increased activation during the moderate processing load condition, but very little increase in activation associated with the highest processing load condition.

Chen et al.[84] utilized the sports concussion research model and fMRI to study cerebral activation patterns associated with working memory after MTBI. Sixteen athletes were studied with fMRI techniques between 1 and 14 months postinjury, using a working memory task with a single processing load. Fifteen of the athletes were symptomatic at the time of study. Activation patterns in a group of control subjects were used to define ROIs, and the degree of activation within the ROIs and extent of activation outside of the ROIs were compared across groups. Although performance on the task did not differ between the groups, the concussed group showed reduced activation in frontal ROIs and increased areas of activation in parietal and temporal regions relative to controls. The researchers concluded that their results demonstrated the potential of fMRI, in conjunction with effective working memory paradigms, to identify the underlying pathology of systematic MTBI patients who otherwise have normal structural imaging results.[84]

Jantzen et al.[85] conducted a prospective fMRI study of MTBI in collegiate football players in which four players who suffered concussion underwent fMRI studies within one week of injury, with results compared to preseason baseline functional imaging studies. When compared with control subjects, concussed players had marked within-subject increases in the amplitude and extent of blood-oxygen-level–dependent activity during a finger-sequencing task, with effects observed primarily in the parietal and lateral frontal and cerebellar regions. Differences in neuronal functioning were observed in the absence of observed differences in behavioral or cognitive performance, which the investigators interpreted as indicating that fMRI techniques may have better sensitivity to concussion compared to neuropsychological evaluation alone in understanding MTBI and identifying mechanisms of recovery.[85]

A 2006 report by McAllister et al.[86] reviewed evidence from fMRI and neurogenetic studies on mechanisms of working memory dysfunction after mild and moderate TBI. They concluded that fMRI in individuals with mild and moderate TBI suggests that they can have problems in the activation and allocation of working memory, and several lines of evidence suggest that subtle alterations in central catecholaminergic sensitivity may underlie these working memory problems. McAllister and colleagues also comment that there is significant evidence for dysfunction of catecholaminergic systems associated with TBI,[86] but less is known about these effects at the milder end of the TBI spectrum. After more severe forms of TBI, circulating levels of dopamine, norepinephrine, and epinephrine may be markers of injury severity and likelihood of recovery, based largely on animal studies.[87,88]

It is also suggested that administration of certain catecholaminergic agents may enhance recovery from brain injury in both animal models and humans.[86] fMRI techniques are now being used to study the effects of catecholaminergic agonists on cognitive functioning after TBI. McAllister et al.[89] specifically studied this concept as it relates to MTBI. Bromocriptine (dopamine D_2 agonist) 1.25 mg or placebo was administered to 12 healthy controls and 16 individuals with mild TBI. They found a significant type of drug-by-diagnosis interaction on the N-back cognitive paradigm in their fMRI study, with the controls showing modest gains in performance that were not seen in the mild TBI group. fMRI activation patterns during this task also showed a significant drug-by-diagnosis interaction indicating a different pattern of drug-induced activation along an anterior–posterior gradient within the frontal lobes. The investigators concluded that these preliminary results suggest that, one month after injury, MTBI subjects and controls showed different responses to dopamine agonists, and these performance differences are associated with different, localized increases in activation of dorsolateral prefrontal cortex during working memory tasks.

Based on a comprehensive review of the literature, McAllister et al.[86] assert that, collectively, fMRI research of MTBI provides evidence consistent with the hypotheses that TBI is associated with dysregulation of allocation of working memory processing resources. Some limitations inherent to fMRI studies, however, require consideration in carefully interpreting results across studies. Nonetheless, several trends in fMRI research are evident.

Though preliminary, fMRI may have greater sensitivity to MTBI than other clinical or neuroimaging techniques, with the capability of advancing our understanding of the natural history of neurophysiologic recovery after MTBI, which is discussed further with presentation of data in chapter 12 on measuring neurophysiologic recovery.

Single-Photon-Emission Computed Tomography (SPECT)

Several studies have attempted to apply SPECT in the study of both acute and chronic MTBI.[90–93] These studies assert that SPECT may be more sensitive than other neuroimaging techniques, based predominately on findings that show abnormalities on SPECT imaging in a high percentage of subjects with normal CT scans. When conducted within the first few weeks postinjury, most SPECT studies reveal hypoperfusion associated with MTBI,[73,94,95] typically in the frontal and temporal lobes known to be preferentially susceptible to the effects of traumatic brain injury. This prevalence has ranged in the order of 60–90 percent. Other studies of MTBI patients who had no CT reported decreased regional cerebral blood flow on SPECT in 61 percent of patients. Similar to other newer imaging techniques, fewer studies have investigated the sensitivity of SPECT in asymptomatic MTBI patient or correlated abnormalities on SPECT with clinical variables and long-term outcome after MTBI.[91]

Positron Emission Tomography (PET)

PET scanning detects blood flow, oxygen, and glucose metabolism, rather than regional blood flow as in the case of SPECT. Very little is known about the sensitivity and specificity of PET in relation to MTBI because existing studies have grouped TBI of all severity levels. Additionally, most studies have applied PET imaging during the chronic stage in patients with persistent post-concussive complaints, rather than during the acute or sub acute postinjury stage.

Hofman et al.[73] studied 21 consecutive MTBI patients (all with GCS scores of 14–15, unconsciousness < 20 min, posttraumatic amnesia < 6 hr) who underwent MRI, SPECT, and neurocognitive assessment within five days after injury. Neurocognitive follow-up was conducted two and six months after injury, and MRI was repeated after six months. Fifty-seven percent of patients had abnormal MRI findings, and 61 percent had abnormal SPECT findings. Additionally, patients with abnormal MRI or SPECT findings had brain atrophy at follow-up, but the mean neurocognitive performance of all subjects was within normal range, and there were no differences in neurocognitive performance between patients with normal and abnormal MRI findings. Seven patients had persistent neurocognitive complaints, and one patient met the criteria for PCS. In total, 77 percent of the MTBI patients had abnormal findings either on MRI or SPECT. Investigators concluded that the association between hypoperfusion seen on acute SPECT and brain atrophy after six months suggested the possibility of (secondary) ischemic brain damage, but there was only a weak correlation between neuroimaging findings and neurocognitive outcome. This study included no control group, however, and therefore, the specificity of these findings remains unclear.

McAllister et al.[82] indicated that several SPECT studies of mixed injury severity suggest that SPECT shows perfusion deficits, some correlating with cognitive deficits in the absence of structural abnormalities on conventional imaging. The ultimate value of PET imaging in MTBI is questionable. While there is suggestion of improved sensitivity of PET over MRI and CT scanning in demonstrating brain dysfunction in the absence of structural abnormalities after MTBI, most PET studies are limited to single case reports or small case series with little or no correlation with neuropsychological test performance or outcome measurement. The sensitivity and specificity of PET at the individual case level also remain unclear from small-group studies.

Conclusion

In summary, CT scanning remains the imaging technique of choice in a critical care setting where the highest priority is to identify any underlying neurosurgical emergency after any form of head trauma, but has the poorest sensitivity in the overwhelming majority of MTBI cases. MRI is more sensitive than CT in demonstrating structural abnormalities after MTBI, and new generations of MRI methods and parameters are enhancing the overall sensitivity of MRI in MTBI, but also have limited utility in predicting long-term outcome. Newer imaging techniques (DTI, MTI, MSI, MRS, fMRI, PET, SPECT) show promise of greater sensitivity than conventional CT and MRI in detecting subtle structural and *functional* abnormalities associated with MTBI. It remains to be seen, however, whether imaging abnormalities in MTBI extend beyond the postacute stage several days to weeks postinjury, or if abnormalities are consistently detectable in asymptomatic MTBI patients.[61] Additional research is also required to demonstrate the ultimate diagnostic utility of these newer methods, as well as correlating imaging findings with quantitative measures of clinical recovery and outcome following MTBI. Belanger et al.[61] appropriately call for prospective studies of both symptomatic and asymptomatic patients to determine the sensitivity, incremental validity, and functional correlates of newer imaging techniques in MTBI.

Part Two Top 10 Conclusions

1. **Scientific advances over the past decade have filled a previously significant void in our direct knowledge of the**

biomechanics, neurophysiology, and functional neuroanatomy of MTBI, which provides a sound and necessary empirical base on which to build our understanding of the true natural history of clinical effects and recovery after MTBI.

2. Several studies using innovative methods have begun to establish a minimal biomechanical threshold sufficient to cause MTBI, which is estimated to be in the range of 80–100g for translational acceleration; the influence of rotational forces must be considered as a mediating factor that may lower the threshold of pure translational force necessary to cause MTBI.

3. In a clinical setting, evidence of a minimal biomechanical threshold for MTBI should be considered when determining if the accident in question was sufficient to cause brain injury and whether the biomechanics correlate with the patient's presenting complaints.

4. Groundbreaking research has now delineated a rather clear pathophysiology of MTBI referred to as the "neurometabolic cascade" and characterized by a stepwise process of ionic shifts, altered brain metabolism, impaired neuronal connectivity, and disruption of normal neurotransmission.

5. The time course of return to normal cerebral function after the metabolic cascade induced by MTBI is not entirely clear, but the bulk of evidence suggests a gradual reversal of physiologic abnormalities and return to normal brain metabolic function within days to weeks after MTBI.

6. The evidence-based time course of physiologic and metabolic recovery after MTBI is strikingly similar to emerging data plotting the true natural history of clinical effects and recovery after MTBI (as reviewed in part three).

7. CT scanning remains the imaging technique of choice in a critical care setting where the highest priority is to identify any underlying neurosurgical emergency after any form of head injury, but has it has the poorest sensitivity in the overwhelming majority of MTBI cases.

8. MRI is more sensitive than CT in demonstrating structural abnormalities after MTBI, and new generations of MRI methods and parameters are enhancing the overall sensitivity of MRI in MTBI.

9. The presence of structural abnormalities on CT and MRI (i.e., complicated MTBI) indicates a more severe gradient of injury relative to uncomplicated MTBI and increases the risk of slow or incomplete recovery after MTBI, but does not provide a perfect predictor of good or poor outcome in the majority of MTBI patients.

10. Emerging neuroimaging technologies may provide greater diagnostic sensitivity than CT and MRI in MTBI, but additional research is required to determine the specificity, incremental validity, and prognostic value of these imaging techniques in measuring recovery and predicting outcome after MTBI.

References

1. Ommaya AK, Gennarelli TA. Cerebral concussion and traumatic unconsciousness. Correlation of experimental and clinical observations of blunt head injuries. *Brain* 1974;97:633–54.

2. Ommaya AK, Gennarelli TA, Thibault LE. Traumatic unconsciousness: mechanisms of brain injury in violent shaking of the head. In: Proceedings of the American Association of Neurological Surgeons; Los Angeles, CA; 1973.

3. Yarnell PR, Lynch S. The 'ding': amnestic states in football trauma. *Neurology* 1973;23:196–97.

4. Yarnell PR, Lynch S. Retrograde memory immediately after concussion. *Lancet* 1970;1:863–64.

5. Ucar T, Tanriover G, Gurer I, Onal MZ, Kazan S. Modified experimental mild traumatic brain injury model. *J Trauma* 2006;60:558–65.

6. Newman JA, Beusenberg M, Fournier E, et al. A new biomechanical assessment of mild traumatic brain injury, part 1: methodology. In:

Proceedings of International Research Conference on the Biomechanics of Impacts; Barcelona, Spain; September 24–25, 1999.

7. Newman JA, Barr C, Beusenberg M, et al. A new biomechanical assessment of mild traumatic brain injury, part 2: results and conclusions. In: Proceedings of International Research Conference on the Biomechanics of Impacts; Montpellier, France; 2000.

8. Pellman EJ, Viano DC, Tucker AM, Casson IR, Waeckerle JF. Concussion in professional football: reconstruction of game impacts and injuries. *Neurosurgery* 2003;53:799–814.

9. Pellman EJ, Viano DC, Tucker AM, Casson IR. Concussion in professional football: location and direction of helmet impacts—part 2. *Neurosurgery* 2003;53:1328–41.

10. Pellman EJ. Background on the National Football League's research on concussion in professional football. *Neurosurgery* 2003;53:797–98.

11. Zhang L, Yang KH, King AI. A proposed injury threshold for mild traumatic brain injury. *J Biomech Eng* 2004;126:226–36.

12. Brolinson PG, Manoogian S, McNeely D, Goforth M, Greenwald R, Duma S. Analysis of linear head accelerations from collegiate football impacts. *Curr Sports Med Rep* 2006;5:23–28.

13. Naunheim RS, Standeven J, Richter C, Lewis LM. Comparison of impact data in hockey, football, and soccer. *J Trauma* 2000;48:938–41.

14. Mihalik JP, Guskiewicz K, Bell DR, et al. Evaluation of impact biomechanics: the association between impact magnitudes and locations in collegiate football players. *J Athl Train* 2006;41:S40–S41.

15. Bell DR, Mihalik JP, Guskiewicz K, et al. An analysis of head impacts sustained during a complete season by Division I collegiate football players. *J Athl Train* 2006;41:S40.

16. McCaffrey MA, Mihalik JP, Guskiewicz K, et al. Balance and neurocognitive performance in collegiate football players following head impacts at varying magnitudes. *J Athl Train* 2006;41:S41.

17. Mihalik JP, Guskiewicz K, Notebaert AJ, et al. Measurement of head impacts in Division I collegiate football players. *J Athl Train* 2005;40:S82.

18. Guskiewicz K, Mihalik JP, Notebaert AJ, et al. Recurrent concussion in a collegiate football player equipped with the Head Impact Telemetry System. *J Athl Train* 2005;40:S81.

19. Guskiewicz K. Personal communication with the author on the biomechanics of sport-related MTBI. Chapel Hill, NC, 2006.

20. Giza CC, Hovda DA. The pathophysiology of traumatic brain injury. In: Lovell MR, Echemendia RJ, Barth JT, Collins MW, ed. *Traumatic Brain Injury in Sports: An International Neuropsychological Perspective.* Exton, PA: Swets & Zeitlinger, 2004:45–70.

21. Shaw NA. The neurophysiology of concussion. *Prog Neurobiol* 2002; 67:281–344.

22. Iverson GL. Outcome from mild traumatic brain injury. *Curr Opin Psychiatry* 2005;18:301–17.

23. Iverson GL, Lange RT, Gaetz M, Zasler ND. Mild TBI. In: Zasler ND, Katz DI, Zafonte RD, ed. *Brain Injury Medicine: Principles and Practice.* New York: Demos Medical Publishing, 2006:333–71.

24. Giza CC, Hovda DA. The neurometabolic cascade of concussion. *J Athl Train* 2001;36:228–35.

25. Gennarelli TA, Graham DI. Neuropathology of the head injuries. *Semin Clin Neuropsychiatry* 1998;3:160–75.

26. Voller B, Auff E, Schnider P, Aichner F. To do or not to do? Magnetic resonance imaging in mild traumatic brain injury. *Brain Inj* 2001;15: 107–15.

27. Yoshino A, Hovda DA, Kawamata T, Katayama Y, Becker DP. Dynamic changes in local cerebral glucose utilization following cerebral conclusion in rats: evidence of a hyper- and subsequent hypometabolic state. *Brain Res* 1991;561:106–19.

28. Cortez SC, McIntosh TK, Noble LJ. Experimental fluid percussion brain injury: vascular disruption and neuronal and glial alterations. *Brain Res* 1989;482:271–82.

29. Fineman I, Hovda DA, Smith M, Yoshino A, Becker DP. Concussive brain injury is associated with a prolonged accumulation of calcium: a 45Ca autoradiographic study. *Brain Res* 1993;624:94–102.

30. McIntosh TK. Novel pharmacologic therapies in the treatment of experimental traumatic brain injury: a review. *J Neurotrauma* 1993;10: 215–61.

31. Osteen CL, Moore AH, Prins ML, Hovda DA. Age-dependency of [45]calcium accumulation following lateral fluid percussion: acute and delayed patterns. *J Neurotrauma* 2001;18:141–62.

32. Hovda DA, Yoshino A, Kawamata T, Katayama Y, Becker DP. Diffuse prolonged depression of cerebral oxidative metabolism following concussive brain injury in the rat: a cytochrome oxidase histochemistry study. *Brain Res* 1991;567:1–10.

33. Gardiner M, Smith ML, Kagstrom E, Shohami E, Siesjo BK. Influence of blood glucose concentration on brain lactate accumulation during severe hypoxia and subsequent recovery of brain energy metabolism. *J Cereb Blood Flow Metab* 1982;2:429–38.

34. Kalimo H, Rehncrona S, Soderfeldt B, Olsson Y, Siesjo BK. Brain lactic acidosis and ischemic cell damage: 2. Histopathology. *J Cereb Blood Flow Metab* 1981;1:313–27.

35. Kalimo H, Rehncrona S, Soderfeldt B. The role of lactic acidosis in the ischemic nerve cell injury. *Acta Neuropathol Suppl* (Berl) 1981; 7:20–2.

36. Myers RE. A unitary theory of causation of anoxic and hypoxic brain pathology. *Adv Neurol* 1979;26:195–213.

37. Siemkowicz E, Hansen AJ. Clinical restitution following cerebral ischemia in hypo-, normo- and hyperglycemic rats. *Acta Neurol Scand* 1978;58:1–8.

38. Bergsneider M, Hovda DA, Lee SM, et al. Dissociation of cerebral glucose metabolism and level of consciousness during the period of metabolic depression following human traumatic brain injury. *J Neurotrauma* 2000;17:389–401.

39. Vink R, McIntosh TK, Demediuk P, Faden AI. Decrease in total and free magnesium concentration following traumatic brain injury in rats. *Biochem Biophys Res Commun* 1987;149:594–99.

40. Vink R, McIntosh TK, Weiner MW, Faden AI. Effects of traumatic brain injury on cerebral high-energy phosphates and pH: a 31P magnetic resonance spectroscopy study. *J Cereb Blood Flow Metab* 1987;7:563–71.

41. Vink R, Faden AI, McIntosh TK. Changes in cellular bioenergetic state following graded traumatic brain injury in rats: determination by phosphorus 31 magnetic resonance spectroscopy. *J Neurotrauma* 1988;5:315–30.

42. Vink R, McIntosh TK. Pharmacological and physiological effects of magnesium on experimental traumatic brain injury. *Magnes Res* 1990;3:163–69.

43. D'Ambrosio R, Maris DO, Grady MS, Winn HR, Janigro D. Selective loss of hippocampal long-term potentiation, but not depression, following fluid percussion injury. *Brain Res* 1998;786:64–79.

44. Sick TJ, Perez-Pinzon MA, Feng ZZ. Impaired expression of long-term potentiation in hippocampal slices 4 and 48 h following mild fluid-percussion brain injury in vivo. *Brain Res* 1998;785:287–92.

45. Sanders MJ, Sick TJ, Perez-Pinzon MA, Dietrich WD, Green EJ. Chronic failure in the maintenance of long-term potentiation following fluid percussion injury in the rat. *Brain Res* 2000;861:69–76.

46. Gorman LK, Fu K, Hovda DA, Murray M, Traystman RJ. Effects of traumatic brain injury on the cholinergic system in the rat. *J Neurotrauma* 1996;13:457–63.

47. Schmidt RH, Grady MS. Loss of forebrain cholinergic neurons following fluid-percussion injury: implications for cognitive impairment in closed head injury. *J Neurosurg* 1995;83:496–502.

48. Ingebrigtsen T, Romner B. Biochemical serum markers for brain damage: a short review with emphasis on clinical utility in mild head injury. *Restor Neurol Neurosci* 2003;21:171–6.

49. Ingebrigtsen T, Romner B. Biochemical serum markers of traumatic brain injury. *J Trauma* 2002;52:798–808.

50. Ingebrigtsen T, Romner B. Serial S-100 protein serum measurements related to early magnetic resonance imaging after minor head injury. Case report. *J Neurosurg* 1996;85:945–48.

51. Mussack T, Biberthaler P, Kanz KG, et al. Immediate S-100B and neuron-specific enolase plasma measurements for rapid evaluation of primary brain damage in alcohol-intoxicated, minor head-injured patients. *Shock* 2002;18:395–400.

52. Biberthaler P, Mussack T, Wiedemann E, et al. Influence of alcohol exposure on S-100b serum levels. *Acta Neurochir Suppl* 2000;76:177–79.

53. Mussack T, Biberthaler P, Kanz KG, et al. Serum S-100B and interleukin-8 as predictive markers for comparative neurologic outcome analysis of patients after cardiac arrest and severe traumatic brain injury. *Crit Care Med* 2002;30:2669–74.

54. de Kruijk JR, Leffers P, Menheere PP, Meerhoff S, Twijnstra A. S-100B and neuron-specific enolase in serum of mild traumatic brain injury

patients. A comparison with health controls. *Acta Neurol Scand* 2001;103:175–79.

55. Herrmann M, Curio N, Jost S, et al. Release of biochemical markers of damage to neuronal and glial brain tissue is associated with short and long term neuropsychological outcome after traumatic brain injury. *J Neurol Neurosurg Psychiatry* 2001;70:95–100.

56. Biberthaler P, Mussack T, Wiedemann E, et al. Evaluation of S-100b as a specific marker for neuronal damage due to minor head trauma. *World J Surg* 2001;25:93–97.

57. Biberthaler P, Mussack T, Wiedemann E, et al. Elevated serum levels of S-100B reflect the extent of brain injury in alcohol intoxicated patients after mild head trauma. *Shock* 2001;16:97–101.

58. Bazarian JJ, Blyth B, Cimpello L. Bench to bedside: evidence for brain injury after concussion—looking beyond the computed tomography scan. *Acad Emerg Med* 2006;13:199–214.

59. Begaz T, Kyriacou DN, Segal J, Bazarian JJ. Serum biochemical markers for post-concussion syndrome in patients with mild traumatic brain injury. *J Neurotrauma* 2006;23:1201–10.

60. Williams DH, Levin HS, Eisenberg HM. Mild head injury classification. *Neurosurgery* 1990;27:422–8.

61. Belanger HG, Vanderploeg RD, Curtiss G, Warden DL. Recent neuroimaging techniques in mild traumatic brain injury. *J Neuropsychiatry Clin Neurosci* 2007;19:5–20.

62. National Center for Health Statistics. 2000 National Hospital Ambulatory Medical Care Survey Micro-Data File Documentation. Vol. 2003. Atlanta, GA: Centers for Disease Control and Prevention, 2003.

63. Jagoda AS, Cantrill SV, Wears RL, et al. Clinical policy: neuroimaging and decisionmaking in adult mild traumatic brain injury in the acute setting. *Ann Emerg Med* 2002;40:231–49.

64. Iverson GL, Lovell MR, Smith S, Franzen MD. Prevalence of abnormal CT-scans following mild head injury. *Brain Inj* 2000;14:1057–61.

65. French BN, Dublin AB. The value of computerized tomography in the management of 1000 consecutive head injuries. *Surg Neurol* 1977;7:171–83.

66. Jeret JS, Mandell M, Anziska B, et al. Clinical predictors of abnormality disclosed by computed tomography after mild head trauma. *Neurosurgery* 1993;32:9–16.

67. Livingston DH, Loder PA, Koziol J, Hunt CD. The use of CT scanning to triage patients requiring admission following minimal head injury. *J Trauma* 1991;31:483–89.

68. Iverson GL, Brooks BL, Collins MW, Lovell MR. Tracking neuropsychological recovery following concussion in sport. *Brain Inj* 2006;20:245–52.

69. Bazarian JJ. Evidence-based emergency medicine. Corticosteroids for traumatic brain injury. *Ann Emerg Med* 2002;40:515–17.

70. Mittl RL, Grossman RI, Hiehle JF, et al. Prevalence of MR evidence of diffuse axonal injury in patients with mild head injury and normal head CT findings. *Am J Neuroradiol* 1994;15:1583–89.

71. Hammoud DA, Wasserman BA. Diffuse axonal injuries: pathophysiology and imaging. *Neuroimaging Clin N Am* 2002;12:205–16.

72. Doezema D, King JN, Tandberg D, Espinosa MC, Orrison WW. Magnetic resonance imaging in minor head injury. *Ann Emerg Med* 1991;20:1281–85.

73. Hofman PA, Stapert SZ, van Kroonenburgh MJ, Jolles J, de Kruijk J, Wilmink JT. MR imaging, single-photon emission CT, and neurocognitive performance after mild traumatic brain injury. *Am J Neuroradiol* 2001;22:441–49.

74. Voller B, Benke T, Benedetto K, Schnider P, Auff E, Aichner F. Neuropsychological, MRI and EEG findings after very mild traumatic brain injury. *Brain Inj* 1999;13:821–27.

75. Hughes DG, Jackson A, Mason DL, Berry E, Hollis S, Yates DW. Abnormalities on magnetic resonance imaging seen acutely following mild traumatic brain injury: correlation with neuropsychological tests and delayed recovery. *Neuroradiology* 2004;46:550–58.

76. Kurca E, Sivak S, Kucera P. Impaired cognitive functions in mild traumatic brain injury patients with normal and pathologic magnetic resonance imaging. *Neuroradiology* 2006;48:661–69.

77. Arfanakis K, Haughton VM, Carew JD, Rogers BP, Dempsey RJ, Meyerand ME. Diffusion tensor MR imaging in diffuse axonal injury. *Am J Neuroradiol* 2002;23:794–802.

78. Inglese M, Makani S, Johnson G, et al. Diffuse axonal injury in mild traumatic brain injury: a diffusion tensor imaging study. *J Neurosurg* 2005;103:298–303.

79. Bagley LJ, McGowan JC, Grossman RI, et al. Magnetization transfer imaging of traumatic brain injury. *J Magn Reson Imaging* 2000;11:1–8.

80. Christodoulou C, DeLuca J, Ricker JH, et al. Functional magnetic resonance imaging of working memory impairment after traumatic brain injury. *J Neurol Neurosurg Psychiatry* 2001;71:161–68.

81. Govindaraju V, Gauger GE, Manley GT, Ebel A, Meeker M, Maudsley AA. Volumetric proton spectroscopic imaging of mild traumatic brain injury. *Am J Neuroradiol* 2004;25:730–37.

82. McAllister TW, Sparling MB, Flashman LA, Saykin AJ. Neuroimaging findings in mild traumatic brain injury. *J Clin Exp Neuropsychol* 2001;23:775–91.

83. McAllister TW, Saykin AJ, Flashman LA, et al. Brain activation during working memory 1 month after mild traumatic brain injury: a functional MRI study. *Neurology* 1999;53:1300–8.

84. Chen JK, Johnston KM, Frey S, Petrides M, Worsley K, Ptito A. Functional abnormalities in symptomatic concussed athletes: an fMRI study. *Neuroimage* 2004;22:68–82.

85. Jantzen KJ, Anderson B, Steinberg FL, Kelso JA. A prospective functional MR imaging study of mild traumatic brain injury in college football players. *Am J Neuroradiol* 2004;25:738–45.

86. McAllister TW, Flashman LA, McDonald BC, Saykin AJ. Mechanisms of working memory dysfunction after mild and moderate TBI: evidence from functional MRI and neurogenetics. *J Neurotrauma* 2006;23: 1450–67.

87. McIntosh TK. Neurochemical sequelae of traumatic brain injury: therapeutic implications. *Cerebrovasc Brain Metab Rev* 1994;6:109–62.

88. McIntosh TK, Juhler M, Wieloch T. Novel pharmacologic strategies in the treatment of experimental traumatic brain injury: 1998. *J Neurotrauma* 1998;15:731–69.

89. McAllister TW, Flashman LA, Shaw PK, et al. Differential activation of working memory-associated frontal cortex using a dopamine agonist after mild traumatic brain injury (MTBI). *J Neuropsychiatry Clin Neurosci* 2003;15:278.

90. Abu-Judeh HH, Parker R, Aleksic S, et al. SPECT brain perfusion findings in mild or moderate traumatic brain injury. *Nucl Med Rev Cent East Eur* 2000;3:5–11.

91. Audenaert K, Jansen HM, Otte A, et al. Imaging of mild traumatic brain injury using 57Co and 99mTc HMPAO SPECT as compared to other diagnostic procedures. *Med Sci Monit* 2003;9:MT112–17.

92. Abu-Judeh HH, Parker R, Singh M, et al. SPET brain perfusion imaging in mild traumatic brain injury without loss of consciousness and normal computed tomography. *Nucl Med Commun* 1999;20:505–10.

93. Abdel-Dayem HM, Abu-Judeh H, Kumar M, et al. SPECT brain perfusion abnormalities in mild or moderate traumatic brain injury. *Clin Nucl Med* 1998;23:309–17.

94. Nedd K, Sfakianakis G, Ganz W, et al. 99mTc-HMPAO SPECT of the brain in mild to moderate traumatic brain injury patients: compared with CT—a prospective study. *Brain Inj* 1993;7:469–79.

95. Umile EM, Plotkin RC, Sandel ME. Functional assessment of mild traumatic brain injury using SPECT and neuropsychological testing. *Brain Inj* 1998;12:577–94.

PART THREE

THE NATURAL HISTORY OF MTBI

Following the progression from delineating the basic science of mild traumatic brain injury (MTBI), the discussion now turns to what is essentially the bread and butter of this book: a review of the latest evidence on the true natural history of clinical effects and recovery after MTBI. The book opened with one basic premise: that determining the true natural history of injury historically has been the greatest challenge facing both clinicians and researchers who professionally work in the area of MTBI. Historically, discussion of "natural history" has typically referred to an end point to long-term recovery. As a neuropsychologist, I am often struck by the fact that my particular specialty is not involved early in the course of MTBI, but then often we are called upon months or even years after injury to determine whether a patient's presenting cognitive or other complaints are likely attributable to a previous MTBI or other factors. Again, the point stressed here is that all things downstream are significantly influenced by their origin and early development, including the course and natural history of MTBI.

Part three reviews the latest research on the natural history of acute and subacute MTBI. Thankfully, several studies over the past 5–10 years have provided data on the early course of recovery in symptoms, cognitive functioning, and other MTBI-related impairments within hours or even minutes of injury. The discussion of recent research on the effects and recovery of MTBI combines a review of several recent meta-analyses focused on MTBI recovery and the results from recent large-scale prospective studies of sport-related concussion. Specifically, part three divided into separate discussions on the course of acute effects and early symptom and cognitive recovery, mid- and long-term neuropsychological recovery, the influence of acute injury characteristics (e.g., loss of consciousness [LOC], posttraumatic amnesia [PTA], structural injury) on recovery, emerging evidence on neurophysiologic recovery, and ultimately the real-life implications of functional outcome after MTBI.

The goal of part three is to integrate findings across these various areas in hopes of informing a consensus on the expected natural history of MTBI. I also discuss possible exceptions to this consensus, particularly in relation to the potential cumulative effects and long-term risks associated with recurrent MTBI.

8

■ ■ ■

Acute Symptoms and Symptom Recovery

As summarized in part one, the diagnosis of MTBI is based in large part on subjective symptoms reported by the patient. Likewise, end points of recovery after MTBI are most often determined by the complete resolution of self-reported symptoms. The diagnosis of postconcussion syndrome (PCS) is essentially reserved for those patients with persistent complaints after MTBI. In sum, the diagnostic and prognostic importance of symptoms after MTBI underscores the need to establish empirically defined parameters for the expected course of symptom recovery. Thankfully, recent studies have generated an evidence base on the natural history of symptom recovery after MTBI that can guide the clinician in interpreting a patient's persistent complaints at the individual case level.

In 2004, the World Health Organization (WHO) Collaborating Centre Task Force on Mild Traumatic Brain Injury published a detailed review of the literature on the prognosis after MTBI. In total, 120 studies of best-evidence synthesis on prognosis after MTBI met their criteria for inclusion in their critical review.[1] Carroll et al. summarize the task force's review:

> There was consistent and methodologically sound evidence that children's prognosis after MTBI is good, with quick resolution of symptoms and little evidence of residual cognitive, behavioral or academic deficits. For adults, cognitive deficits and symptoms are common in the acute stage, and the majority of studies report recovery for most within 3–12 months. Where symptoms persist, compensation and litigation is a factor, but there is little consistent evidence for other predictors. The literature on this area is of

varying quality and causal inferences are often mistakenly drawn from cross sectional studies.[1]

In both children and adults, symptoms after MTBI are typically transient in nature, with rapid or gradual resolution within days to weeks postinjury in an overwhelming majority of MTBI patients.[1] Furthermore, MTBI symptoms are highly nonspecific and often are similar to those reported after other types of injury (e.g., orthopedic injury), as discussed further in part four with respect to the nonspecificity of PCS symptoms.

The WHO task force summarized the results of several studies on self-reported symptoms after MTBI, indicating that headache, blurred vision, dizziness, subjective memory problems, and other cognitive difficulties and sleep problems are the most commonly experienced symptoms after MTBI.[2–12] Most studies indicate a pattern of gradual symptom recovery within the first one to two weeks after MTBI in the overwhelming majority of cases, extending out to several weeks in some instances. Contrary to previous reports, a very small percentage of cases have symptoms persisting beyond three months after MTBI, which is discussed further within the summary on PCS in part four.

In more severe forms of complicated MTBI, focal, structural damage detected on head computed tomography (CT) or brain magnetic resonance imaging (MRI) may increase the risk of slower recovery with prolonged symptoms and poorer overall outcome more consistent that seen in moderately severe TBI.

With respect to uncomplicated MTBI with no structural injury visualized on neuroimaging, however, Carroll et al.[1] summarize the literature on MTBI symptom recovery by stating that there is evidence that persistent symptoms beyond the typical recovery period of several days to weeks may be attributable to factors other than MTBI. Demographic (e.g., female gender, older age), psychosocial (e.g., unstable relationships, lack of social support system, preexisting psychiatric problems or personality disorder, chemical dependency), medical (e.g., severe associated injuries, comorbid medical or neurologic disorders, prior history of MTBI), and situational (e.g., litigation/compensation, concurrent posttraumatic stress disorder) have also been implicated as predictors of prolonged symptoms after MTBI.[1] In one study, Landre et al.[13] reported that hospitalized MTBI patients did not differ from general trauma subjects in their report of postconcussive symptoms five days postinjury and that, when present, persistent symptoms were consistently related to emotional distress.

There is also consistent evidence of a relationship between litigation/compensation and protracted symptom recovery after MTBI. In a meta-analysis of 17 studies, Binder and Rohling[14] reported that financial compensation was a strong risk factor for long-term symptoms and disability after MTBI. Paniak et al.[15,16] also reported that compensation seeking strongly predicted persistent symptoms and poorer functional outcome (e.g., return to work), independent of MTBI severity based on acute injury characteristics.

Prospective Studies of Symptom Recovery

Over the past decade, there has been a significant movement in the neurosciences and other areas of medicine toward the development of various standardized methods for the evaluation of acute MTBI, beyond the classic approach of Glasgow Coma Scale (GCS) and other measures more appropriate for the classification of moderate and severe TBI. This movement has included standardization of various "symptom checklists" that survey a patient's various signs and symptoms of MTBI. These scales not only allow clinicians and researchers to quantify the severity of symptoms, but also lend to *measuring* any change in symptoms during the first several days and weeks postinjury, which is required to plot the natural course of eventual symptom recovery over time.

Our research group has compiled extensive data from three multicenter studies of sport-related concussion that capitalize on the advantages of the sports concussion research module described in part one. Box 8.1 provides an overview of three large, multicenter prospective studies directed by our research group, the NCAA Concussion Study, Project Sideline, and Concussion Prevention Initiative (CPI), that have generated an abundance of evidence on the acute effects and natural recovery course relating to symptoms, cognitive functioning, and other functional deficits following MTBI.

Table 8.1 provides an overview of the injury characteristics documented in the clinical samples from the NCAA Concussion Study, Project Sideline, and CPI. While these three large studies have enabled us to look at several aspects of MTBI effects and management, the principle aim was to prospectively measure the natural course relating to symptoms, cognitive functioning, postural stability, and other effects following sport-related concussion. The ultimate goal is to then compare results from the sports concussion research platform to those in the general MTBI population to determine the generalizability of these findings and the ultimate merit of the sports concussion research model for determining the true natural history of MTBI from any cause.

BOX 8.1 Description of NCAA Concussion Study, Concussion Prevention Initiative, and Project Sideline

Overview

The NCAA Concussion Study (4,251 college player seasons studied) was sponsored by the National Collegiate Athletic Association. The Concussion Prevention Initiative (CPI) (9,094 high school and college player seasons) was sponsored by the National Center for Injury Prevention and Control at the Centers for Disease Control and Prevention and coordinated out of the Injury Prevention Research Center at the University of North Carolina at Chapel Hill. Project Sideline (3,279 high school player seasons) studied high school athletes in suburban Milwaukee, Wisconsin.

Sample

The total sample averaged 17.49 (SD = 1.62) years of age, 10.14 (SD = 1.06) years of education, and 6.72 (SD = 2.86) years of organized participation in the sport being studied. The sample was 88.5 percent male; most concussions studied were in football (80 percent), followed by soccer (13 percent), lacrosse (6 percent), and hockey (1 percent). One-third of subjects (33.5 percent) reported a prior history of concussion, including 6.3 percent with two and 3.1 percent with three or more previous concussions.

Study Design

All players underwent a preseason baseline evaluation on a battery of concussion assessment measures. Injured subjects were identified and enrolled in the study protocol by a team physician or certified athletic trainer present on the sideline during an athletic contest or practice. *Concussion* was defined according to the American Academy of Neurology Guideline for Management of Sports Concussion.[15,19]

The Graded Symptom Checklist (GSC), Balance Error Scoring System (BESS), Standardized Assessment of Concussion (SAC), and a neuropsychological test battery were used to assess postconcussive symptoms, postural stability, and cognitive functioning. Several

(*continued*)

studies on the effects of sport-related concussion have demonstrated the reliability and accuracy of these measures in correctly classifying injured and noninjured subjects after sport-related concussion.[3,4,20–22] Subjects were tested on the GSC, SAC, and BESS on the sideline immediately following injury, 2–3 hr later, and again on several days during the first week postinjury. Neuropsychological testing was administered one to two days and one week postinjury. All measures were then readministered 45 days postinjury (Project Sideline) or 90 days postinjury (NCAA study, CPI). Clinicians also recorded detailed information on acute injury characteristics (e.g., unconsciousness, amnesia), recovery course, symptom-free waiting period (SFWP), incidence of repeat concussion, and other aspects of clinical management in each case.

The design for each of the three studies varied slightly. The NCAA study and CPI study both involved a multiple-arm design stratified based on the intensity of the assessment protocol, from one of the following: (1) routine clinical exam plus the GSC, (2) use of a brief screening battery (GSC, SAC, and BESS), or (3) brief screening battery plus neuropsychological test battery. Participating institutions were randomly assigned to a specific arm of the study, so all injured athletes from that institution underwent the same assessment protocol. Project Sideline was a single group design in which all assessment instruments were used.

Our research group has collected extensive data on symptom recovery beginning within minutes of injury and following the course of symptom recovery out several weeks and months post-MTBI in a large sample of athletes with sport-related concussion. In doing so, we have utilized the Graded Symptom Checklist (GSC) (see Figure 8.1), which is an inventory of common postconcussive symptoms that the subject rates in severity on a 0 to 6 Likert scale adapted from previous postconcussion symptom scales.[17] This instrument not only provides quantitative information on which symptoms are endorsed and their severity, but also then tallies to a composite score that serves as the sturdiest indicator of overall symptom severity, against which to track subsequent recovery.

Table 8.1 Injury Characteristics for NCAA Concussion Study, Concussion Prevention Initiative, and Project Sideline

	NCAA CONCUSSION STUDY	CONCUSSION PREVENTION INITIATIVE (CPI)	PROJECT SIDELINE	TOTAL
Teams	25	124	20	169
Player Seasons	4,251	9,094	3,279	16,624
MTBIs Studied	196	375	87	658
MTBI Severity[a]	%	%	%	
AAN Grade 1–2	93.2	80.7	82.1	90.3
AAN Grade 3	6.8	9.3	17.9	9.7
Acute Injury Characteristics	%	%	%	
LOC	6.8	9.3	17.9	9.7
PTA	19.1	21.9	37.3	22.9
RGA	7.4	17.3	29.9	15.6
No LOC or Amnesia	78.1	64.5	49.4	66.5

Abbreviations: AAN, American Academy of Neurology; LOC, loss of consciousness; PTA, posttraumatic amnesia; RGA, retrograde amnesia.
[a]AAN grade 1 based on alteration of mental status and symptoms resolving within 15 min; AAN grade 2 based on symptoms and abnormalities persisting beyond 15 min, but with no loss of consciousness; AAN grade 3 based on any loss of consciousness (see box 3.5 for AAN grading scale).

Figure 8.2 plots the course of symptom recovery (relative to preinjury baseline) beginning immediately after injury and tracked over the next several hours, days, and weeks after MTBI. Several important points require emphasis. First, as would be intuitively expected, symptomatology is most severe immediately following injury. Second, a pattern of symptom recovery is evident within the first 2 hr of concussion, based on a reduction in total symptom severity score. Furthermore, this pattern of symptom recovery continues on a gradual course over the first several days, such that there is no significant difference between the symptom scores for injured subjects and normal controls by seven days postinjury. Finally, the pattern of symptom recovery is essentially identical in separate populations of high school and college subjects.

Please read the following list of symptoms to the player and indicate if s/he is currently experiencing any of the symptoms. This form should be completed for the injured and control subject.

If the player is <u>not</u> experiencing the symptom, circle the 0 under the "None" column for that symptom.

If the player is currently experiencing the symptom, please indicate how severe the symptoms is by circling the appropriate number on a scale from 1 (very mild) to 6 (very severe).

Symptom	None	Mild		Moderate		Severe	
1. HEADACHE	0	1	2	3	4	5	6
2. NAUSEA (SICK TO STOMACH)	0	1	2	3	4	5	6
3. VOMITING (THROWING UP)	0	1	2	3	4	5	6
4. TEETH HURTING	0	1	2	3	4	5	6
5. BALANCE PROBLEMS/DIZZINESS	0	1	2	3	4	5	6
6. FATIGUE	0	1	2	3	4	5	6
7. SKIN RASH/ITCHING	0	1	2	3	4	5	6
8. TROUBLE SLEEPING	0	1	2	3	4	5	6
9. SLEEPING MORE THAN USUAL	0	1	2	3	4	5	6
10. DROWSINESS (FEELING TIRED)	0	1	2	3	4	5	6
11. SENSITIVITY TO LIGHT	0	1	2	3	4	5	6
12. BLURRED VISION	0	1	2	3	4	5	6
13. SENSITIVITY TO NOISE	0	1	2	3	4	5	6
14. JOINT STIFFNESS (E.G. FINGERS)	0	1	2	3	4	5	6
15. SADNESS	0	1	2	3	4	5	6
16. NERVOUSNESS	0	1	2	3	4	5	6
17. IRRITABILITY	0	1	2	3	4	5	6
18. BURNING FEELING IN FEET	0	1	2	3	4	5	6
19. NUMBNESS/TINGLING	0	1	2	3	4	5	6
20. FEELING SLOWED DOWN	0	1	2	3	4	5	6
21. FEELING LIKE "IN A FOG"	0	1	2	3	4	5	6
22. DIFFICULTY CONCENTRATING	0	1	2	3	4	5	6
23. DIFFICULTY REMEMBERING	0	1	2	3	4	5	6
24. NECK PAIN	0	1	2	3	4	5	6
25. OTHER	0	1	2	3	4	5	6
Column Total Score							

Total # of Items Endorsed	
Overall Total Score	

Assuming you were at 100% before your concussion, give a rating for what percentage you are at now in terms of your overall condition (enter a number between 0 and 100): _____%

FIGURE 8.1. Graded Symptom Checklist. Adapted from Lovell and Collins[17] with permission.

In addition to delineating the group recovery illustrated in Figure 8.2, it is important for the clinician treating the individual MTBI case to have some index of the distribution of recovery rates from large group studies. Table 8.2 categorizes the rate of symptom recovery (relative to individual preinjury baseline symptom score) for subjects in the NCAA, CPI, and Project Sideline studies. Overall, more than 85 percent of injured subjects reported full symptom recovery in less than one week, including 21 percent who reportedly recovered within the first day. Fewer than 3 percent of subjects reported

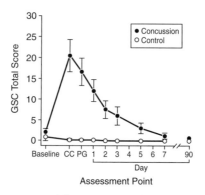

FIGURE 8.2. Symptom recovery following MTBI. Higher scores on the GSC indicate more severe symptoms. Error bars indicate 95% confidence intervals. Baseline is preinjury. CC, time of concussion; PG, postgame/postpractice. Adapted from McCrea et al.[21] with permission.

symptoms beyond one month postinjury, which is considerably lower than previous reports of persistent PCS incidence rates, on the order of 15 percent,[18] that is discussed in part four.

There are also somewhat surprising findings in the distribution of specific symptoms following MTBI. Recent research has demonstrated, for example, that "classic" signs of TBI are rarely observed in the case of MTBI. Figure 8.3

Table 8.2 Distribution of Postinjury Symptom Recovery Course* [% (n)]

CATEGORY OF POSTINJURY SYMPTOM RECOVERY	NCAA	CPI	PROJECT SIDELINE	TOTAL
Rapid (< 1 day)	28.3 (53)	17.4 (64)	21.0 (17)	21.1 (134)
Gradual (> 1 day, < 7 days)	60.4 (113)	68.1 (250)	55.6 (45)	64.3 (408)
Prolonged (1 week to 1 month)	9.6 (18)	11.7 (43)	18.5 (15)	11.9 (76)
Persistent (> 1 month)	1.6 (3)	2.7 (10)	4.9 (4)	2.7 (17)

*Based on documentation from physicians and athletic trainers on duration of symptoms.

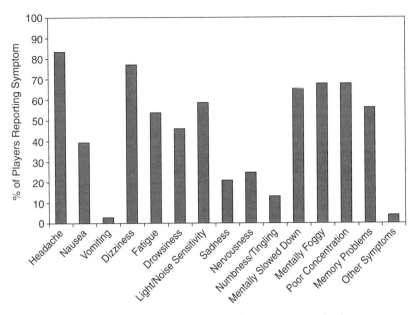

FIGURE 8.3. Frequency of athletes reporting specific symptoms immediately after MTBI.

indicates the percentage of MTBI subjects endorsing various symptoms immediately after injury. During this most acute period, headache, dizziness, sensitivity to light, and a combination of cognitive symptoms (feeling mentally slowed down, mental fogginess, poor concentration, and memory difficulties) are the most frequently reported symptoms.

In contrast, symptoms such as nausea and vomiting, often considered the "red flags" to watch out for in detecting concussion, are much less common. In fact, any occurrence of vomiting was extremely rare. Figures 8.4 and 8.5 illustrate a similar distribution of symptoms, but significantly lower endorsement rates, three and seven days out from injury. Headache is the symptom that most frequently lingers the longest, but is still observed in only about 10 percent of all injured subjects by day 7 postinjury. Overall, 85 percent of subjects report a full symptom recovery within one week and 97 percent within one month.

While select studies have reported longer symptom recovery rates in the non-sport-related MTBI, our findings are quite consistent with the aforementioned WHO conclusions on the general MTBI symptom literature. Studies of sport-related concussion may actually provide a truer measure of

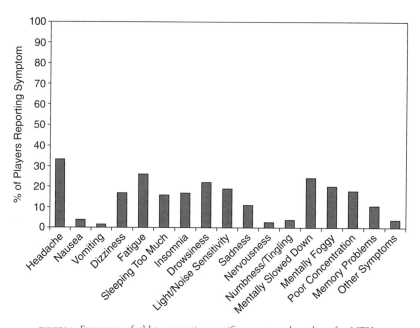

FIGURE 8.4. Frequency of athletes reporting specific symptoms three days after MTBI.

symptom recovery because they most often do not encounter comorbid psychological disorders, adverse motivational factors, possible malingering, and other non-injury-related factors often implicated in the maintenance of postconcussive symptoms in the general MTBI population, particularly those involved in litigation, disability claims, or other similar contexts.

Furthermore, it has been argued that the motivation of the injured athlete is perhaps in the opposite direction of that often observed in the general clinical MTBI population. Most athletes are highly motivated to return to sport participation as soon as possible and therefore are sometimes presumed to underreport symptoms and overestimate their symptom recovery in hopes of an earlier return to competition. At the highest level, professional athletes could also be at risk for significant financial *loss* should persistent symptoms or other difficulties from concussion interrupt their participation or even prompt the need for early retirement from professional sports, as opposed to financial settlement for persistent symptoms or deficits in the context of the general MTBI population.

In a sports setting, this issue indicates the need to correlate symptom recovery with prospective measurement of recovery on standardized performance measures. Athletes may be less than forthcoming about their true symptoms

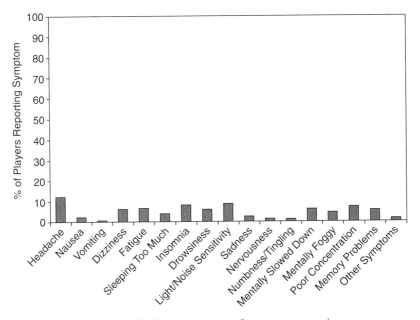

FIGURE 8.5. Frequency of athletes reporting specific symptoms seven days after MTBI.

after concussion but cannot "fake good" in order to exaggerate their recovery on cognitive or other functional measures relative to their own preinjury baseline. Therein lies the value of brief screening instruments and neuropsychological testing to measure cognitive recovery both early and further out from injury. Chapters 9 and 10, however, illustrate that there is almost complete overlap in symptom and cognitive recovery after MTBI: cognitive deficits on standardized testing are infrequently detected in asymptomatic MTBI patients.

Conclusion

In summary, an exhaustive review of the literature and more recent findings from several recent large-scale prospective studies demonstrate several important points relative to natural course of acute symptoms and recovery after MTBI:

- Most severe symptoms are evident within minutes of injury.
- Delayed symptom onset is relatively rare.
- A combination of physical and cognitive symptoms is most common.

Acute Symptoms and Symptom Recovery   95

- Classic signs and symptoms, such as nausea and vomiting, are actually quite rare.
- There is measurable improvement in symptoms within hours of injury.
- A gradual symptom recovery occurs over a period of 7–10 days in an overwhelming majority (80–90 percent) of cases.
- Children and adults show a similar rate and course of symptom recovery.
- More severe forms of complicated MTBI may be at risk of slower recovery and prolonged symptoms.
- Headache is the symptom that tends to linger the longest and to be most problematic in terms of clinical management.
- Symptoms persisting beyond the expected recovery course after MTBI are highly nonspecific to MTBI and are often attributable to non-injury-related factors.

9

■ ■ ■

Acute Cognitive Effects and Early Recovery

Although the persistent cognitive effects of MTBI weeks and months after injury have been extensively researched, relatively fewer studies more recently have provided objective, empirical data on the acute neurocognitive effects immediately following MTBI. This gap in the literature is due in large part to situational circumstances that limit the capacity for prospective research implementing standardized assessment methods immediately following MTBI. Standardized measures for assessing mental status and neurologic changes beyond traditional injury classification criteria (e.g., GCS) are quite uncommon in most trauma settings. Furthermore, injury severity grading systems may not be sensitive to subtle neurocognitive changes that present risks for more severe underlying neurologic complications after MTBI. In contrast, neuropsychological testing is considered a sensitive and sophisticated method for assessing concussion but typically is not feasible immediately after injury in most acute care settings.

Cognitive Screening Tools

Similar to the development of checklists to systematically assess symptoms following MTBI (see chapter 8), the standardization movement has resulted in the development of various objective-screening instruments to quantifiably measure the acute cognitive effects of MTBI. The use of standardized assessment measures allows us not only to reliably and validly detect cognitive impairments that assist the clinician in the diagnoses of MTBI, but also to provide an anchor point against which to quantitatively measure and track recovery over the first several hours, days, and weeks postinjury, particularly when more extensive neuropsychological testing is not feasible.

NAME: _____

TEAM: _____ EXAMINER: _____
DATE OF EXAM: _____ TIME: _____
EXAM (Circle One): BLINE   INJURY   POST-GAME
    FOLLOW-UP DAY: _____

INTRODUCTION:
I am going to ask you some questions.
Please listen carefully and give your best effort.

ORIENTATION

What Month is it? _____	0	1
What's the Date today? _____	0	1
What's the Day of Week? _____	0	1
What Year is it? _____	0	1
What Time is it right now? (within 1 hr.) _____	0	1

Award 1 point for each correct answer

ORIENTATION TOTAL SCORE ➡ [ ]

IMMEDIATE MEMORY

I am going to test your memory. I will read you a list of words and when I am done, repeat back as many words as you can remember, in any order.

List	TRIAL 1	TRIAL 2	TRIAL 3
ELBOW	0 1	0 1	0 1
APPLE	0 1	0 1	0 1
CARPET	0 1	0 1	0 1
SADDLE	0 1	0 1	0 1
BUBBLE	0 1	0 1	0 1
TOTAL			

Trials 2 & 3: I am going to repeat that list again. Repeat back as many words as you can remember in any order, even if you said the word before.

Complete all 3 trials regardless of score on trial 1 & 2. 1 pt. for each correct response. Total score equals sum across all 3 trials.

Do not inform the subject that delayed recall will be tested.

IMMEDIATE MEMORY TOTAL SCORE ➡ [ ]

EXERTIONAL MANEUVERS:

If subject is not displaying or reporting symptoms, conduct the following maneuvers to create conditions under which symptoms likely to be elicited and detected. These measures need to be conducted if a subject is already displaying or reporting any symptoms. If not conducted, allow 2 minutes to keep time delay constant before testing Delayed Recall. These methods should be administered for baseline testing of normal subjects.

EXERTIONAL MANEUVERS	
5 Jumping Jacks	5 Push-Ups
5 Sit-ups	5 Knee Bends

SEE REVERSE SIDE FOR IMPORTANT USER WARNINGS

NEUROLOGIC SCREENING

LOSS OF CONCIOUSNESS/ **WITNESSED UNRESPONSIVENESS**	☐ No Length:	☐ Yes
POST-TRAUMATIC AMNESIA? Poor recall of events after injury	☐ No Length:	☐ Yes
RETROGRADE AMNESIA? Poor recall of events before injury	☐ No Length:	☐ Yes

	NORMAL	ABNORMAL
STRENGTH- Right Upper Extremity	☐	☐
Left Upper Extremity	☐	☐
Right Lower Extremity	☐	☐
Left Lower Extremity	☐	☐
SENSATION - examples: FINGER-TO-NOSE/ROMBERG	☐	☐
COORDINATION - examples: TANDEM WALK/FINGER-NOSE-FINGER	☐	☐

CONCENTRATION

Digits Backward: I am going to read you a string of numbers and when I am done, you repeat them back to me backwards, in reverse order of how I read them to you. For example, if I say 7-1-9, you would say 9-1-7.

If correct, go to next string length. If incorrect, read trial 2. 1 pt. possible for each string length. Stop after incorrect on both trials.

4-9-3	6-2-9	0 1
3-8-1-4	3-2-7-9	0 1
6-2-9-7-1	1-5-2-8-6	0 1
7-1-8-4-6-2	5-3-9-1-4-8	0 1

Months in Reverse Order: Now tell me the months of the year in reverse order. Start with the last month and go backward. So you'll say December, November...Go ahead. 1 pt. for entire sequence correct.

Dec-Nov-Oct-Sept-Aug-Jul-Jun-May-Apr-Mar-Feb-Jan   0   1

CONCENTRATION TOTAL SCORE ➡ [ ]

DELAYED RECALL

Do you remember that list of words I read a few times earlier? Tell me as many words from the list as you can remember in any order. Circle each word correctly recalled. Total score equals number of words recalled.

ELBOW   APPLE   CARPET   SADDLE   BUBBLE

DELAYED RECALL TOTAL SCORE ➡ [ ]

SAC SCORING SUMMARY

Exertional Maneuvers & Neurologic Screening are important for examination, but not incorporated into SAC Total Score.

ORIENTATION	/ 5
IMMEDIATE MEMORY	/ 15
CONCENTRATION	/ 5
DELAYED RECALL	/ 5
SAC TOTAL SCORE ➡	/30

FIGURE 9.1. Standardized Assessment of Concussion (SAC). From McCrea et al.[19] with permission.

The most extensively studied of the cognitive screening tools has been the Standardized Assessment of Concussion (SAC) (see Figure 9.1).[19] The SAC was initially designed according to the recommendations of the American Academy of Neurology (AAN) practice parameter[20] as a brief mental status and neurologic screening instrument to provide sports medicine clinicians with a standardized method of assessing athletes within minutes of having sustained MTBI during competition. Several constraints unfamiliar to traditional neuropsychological testing in a clinical setting were confronted in developing the SAC, including the need for the instrument to be feasible for use on the sport sideline, require minimal training, and meet the psychometric rigors of reliability, validity, sensitivity, and specificity.

Several studies over the past decade have reported on the reliability, validity, sensitivity, and specificity of the SAC as a measure of cognitive functioning following MTBI. More recent studies have illustrated the benefit of the SAC in measuring recovery after MTBI and, more important, informed us as to the natural history of cognitive effects and recovery following MTBI.[21]

In a 2001 study, Barr and McCrea[22] generated reliable change indices (RCI) and multiple regression models computed on retest scores obtained from 68 noninjured athletes who were readministered the SAC either 60 or 120 days following baseline testing. Receiver operating characteristic curve analyses were used to test these models with data obtained on 50 athletes tested immediately following concussion. The results indicated that a decline of one point on the SAC at retesting (postinjury for MTBI group, retest for controls) correctly classified injured and noninjured participants with a level of 94 percent sensitivity and 76 percent specificity (see Table 9.1). The RCI and multiple regression models provided comparable levels of group classification. As expected, detecting clinically meaningful change from individual preinjury baseline score afforded maximum sensitivity and specificity, but this study also generated cutoff scores that are conservative for use with a general MTBI population where baseline data are not available.

Slope of Early Cognitive Recovery

A 2003 study by McCrea et al.[21] illustrated the natural course of early recovery in cognitive functioning based on SAC performance during the first several days following concussion in a large sample of college football players. A prospective cohort of 1,631 collegiate football players were enrolled, and 94 players with concussion (based on the AAN criteria) and 56 noninjured

Table 9.1 Distribution of Observed Differences Between SAC Scores from Time 1 and Time 2

DIFFERENCE SCORE (T1-T2)	TEST-RETEST CONTROL (NUMBER)	ATHLETES WITH CONCUSSION (NUMBER)	SENSITIVITY (SP)	SPECIFICITY (SE)	SUM (SE + SP)
+2	10	0	1.00	.04	1.04
+1	22	0	1.00	.15	1.15
0	20	3	1.00	.53	1.53
−1	5	5	.94	.76	1.70
−2	7	6	.84	.84	1.68
−3	3	9	.72	.93	1.65
−4	1	10	.54	.98	1.52
−5	0	17	.34	1.00	1.34

From Bar and McCrea[22] with permission.

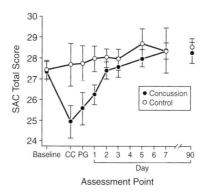

FIGURE 9.2. Cognitive recovery after MTBI. Lower scores on the SAC indicate more severe cognitive impairment. Error bars indicate 95% confidence intervals. Baseline is preinjury. CC, time of concussion; PG, postgame/postpractice. Adapted from McCrea et al.[21] with permission.

controls underwent assessment of symptoms, cognitive functioning, and postural stability immediately, 3 hr, and 1, 2, 3, 5, 7, and 90 days after injury.

Figure 9.2 compares the total SAC score for MTBI subjects and noninjured controls at preinjury baseline testing, immediately following injury, and at several time points over the ensuing hours, days, and weeks after concussion. The pattern of cognitive recovery is highly similar to the resolution of symptoms. That is, the most severe cognitive dysfunction was evident immediately following concussion, but there is already a slope of improvement in cognitive functioning within the first 2–3 hr, which continued on a gradual course over the next several days. There was no significant difference between SAC performance by MTBI subjects and noninjured controls by day two postinjury.

This was reported as the first prospective human study to include preinjury cognitive and motor baseline testing and to plot continuous recovery curves from a point immediately after concussion to several months after injury in a sizable group of humans with concussion. The pattern of impairment exhibited by injured players in the NCAA Concussion Study provided indirect evidence of acute effects and recovery in humans through detailed testing of cognitive functioning, postural stability (see Figure 9.3), and subjective symptoms at serial time points following concussion that match closely the results of animal studies demonstrating a cascade of physiologic events that adversely affect cerebral functioning for period of days to weeks after

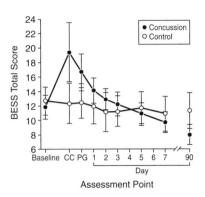

FIGURE 9.3. Postural stability recovery after MTBI. BESS, Balance Error Scoring System. Higher scores on the BESS indicate more severe balance problems. Error bars indicate 95% confidence intervals. Baseline is preinjury. CC indicates time of concussion; PG, postgame/postpractice. Adapted from McCrea et al.[21] with permission.

concussion. In this study, injured athletes exhibited significantly increased symptoms and functional impairment during the acute postconcussive phase that gradually resolved along the same neurophysiologic course described in the animal concussion models (see Figure 9.4).[23]

Individual Rates of Cognitive Recovery

A later study[24] applied standard regression-based methods to statistically measure individual rates of impairment and recovery at several time points after MTBI, including use of the SAC to assess gross cognitive functioning (see Figure 9.5). In this study, acute cognitive dysfunction, as measured by impairment of the SAC, was evident in 80 percent of the injured sample at time of concussion. Persistent cognitive impairment was seen on the SAC in 31 percent of the injured sample on day 1, 23 percent on day 2, and 9 percent (essentially at control levels) on day 7. Statistically defined abnormality on the SAC ranged from only 5 percent to 9 percent of the control group across all assessment points. The SAC had peak sensitivity value of 0.80 at the time of injury and specificity values ranging from 0.89 to 0.98 through day 7.

The SAC and other brief screening instruments are most sensitive and specific in accurately detecting impairments during the acute postinjury phase but have declining sensitivity in detecting more subtle impairments further out from injury (see Table 9.2). In this study, the SAC and more

Mild Traumatic Brain Injury and Postconcussion Syndrome

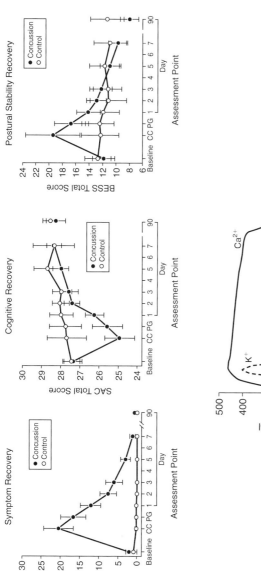

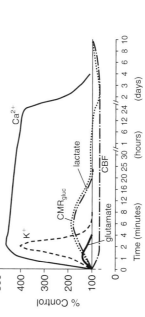

FIGURE 9.4 Comparison of curves for recovery of symptoms, cognitive functioning, and postural stability after MTBI. Higher scores on the GSC indicate more severe symptoms. Lower scores on the SAC indicate more severe cognitive dysfunction. Higher scores on the Balance Error Scoring System (BESS) indicate more severe balance problems. Error bars indicate 95% confidence intervals. Baseline is preinjury. CC, time of concussion, PG, postgame/postpractice. From McCrea et al.[21] and Giza and Hovda[23] with permission.

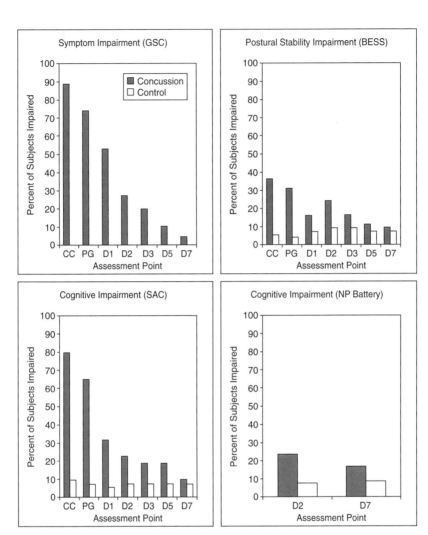

FIGURE 9.5. Percentage of concussion and control subjects classified as impaired based on symptoms, cognitive dysfunction, and postural stability problems from time of injury through day 7. BESS, Balance Error Scoring System; NP Battery, neuropsychological test battery. Assessment Points: CC, time of concussion; PG, postgame/postpractice; D1, postinjury day 1; D2, postinjury day 2, etc. From McCrea et al.[24] with permission.

extensive neuropsychological test battery yielded similar rates of impairment on day 2, but neuropsychological testing provided a more sensitive measure of subtle cognitive dysfunction further out from injury, characterized by mild residual deficits and delayed recall memory, cognitive processing speed, and verbal fluency (see Figure 9.6).

Mild Traumatic Brain Injury and Postconcussion Syndrome

Table 9.2 Sensitivity (Se) and Specificity (Sp) for Detecting Impairment at Postinjury Time Points

	TIME OF INJURY		POST-GAME		DAY 1		DAY 2		DAY 3		DAY 5		DAY 7	
	SE	SP	SE	SP	SE	SP	SE	SP	SE	SP	SE	SP	SE	SP
GSC	.89	1.00	.74	1.00	.53	1.00	.27	1.00	.20	1.00	.10	1.00	.04	1.00
BESS	.34	.91	.32	.96	.16	.93	.24	.91	.16	.91	.10	.93	.07	.95
SAC	.80	.91	.65	.93	.31	.95	.22	.89	.18	.93	.18	.93	.02	.98
Brief Battery Without NP Testing	.94	.89	.86	.89	.69	.89	.51	.84	.38	.84	.26	.87	.14	.93
NP Testing							.23	.93					.19	.91
Full Battery With NP Testing							.56	.79					.30	.86

Reprinted from McCrea et al.[24] with permission.

GSC, Graded Symptom Checklist[17]; BESS, Balance Error Scoring System (Guskiewicz et al. 2001)[114]; SAC, Standardized Assessment of Concussion[19]; NP Testing, neuropsychological test battery. Sensitivity (Se) values indicate the probability that a player originally injured continued to be correctly classified as "abnormal." Specificity (Sp) refers to the probability that a control subject will be correctly classified as "normal" using the same method.

[a]Brief battery refers to GSC, BESS, and SAC.

[b]Full battery refers to brief battery plus neuropsychological testing.

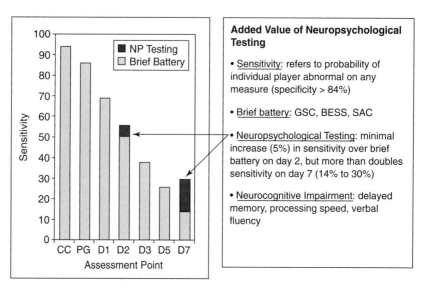

FIGURE 9.6. Incremental value of neuropsychological testing after sport-related MTBI. BESS, Balance Error Scoring System; NP Battery, neuropsychological test battery. Assessment Points: CC, time of concussion; PG, postgame/postpractice; D1, postinjury day 1; D2, postinjury day 2, etc. Adapted from McCrea et al.[24] with permission.

Interval Value of Cognitive Assessment

This study by McCrea et al[24] also allowed investigation of the interval value of neuropsychological testing in detecting impairments in MTBI subjects who otherwise reported a complete symptom recovery. In a sports context, this is especially critical given that these subjects, based on their reported symptom recovery, would otherwise be considered for clearance to return to competition. Ultimately, standardized measures should provide clinicians with a method for detecting impairments in the subject that is otherwise reporting to be symptom free.

Table 9.3 illustrates the percentage of asymptomatic MTBI participants classified as "impaired" (relative to their own personal preinjury baseline) on the Balance Error Scoring System (BESS)[114], SAC, and neuropsychological test battery two days and seven days post-MTBI, compared to the rate of impairment in matched noninjured controls (false-positive rate). With respect to cognitive functioning, the SAC and neuropsychological test battery have similar sensitivity two days postinjury, but the neuropsychological test battery has superior sensitivity further out from injury. The figure of 16 percent of

Table 9.3 Percentage of Asymptomatic Subjects After Concussion (Sx−) and Control Subjects Classified as "Impaired" on Postinjury Days 2 and 7

	DAY 2		DAY 7	
	SX− IMPAIRED (%) (N = 68)	CONTROL IMPAIRED (%) (N = 56)	SX− IMPAIRED (%) (N = 85)	CONTROL IMPAIRED (%) (N = 56)
BESS	37	9	8	7
SAC	16	7	7	7
NP Battery	15	8	16	9

Reprinted from McCrea et al.[24] with permission.
BESS, Balance Error Scoring System (Guskiewicz et al., 2001)[114]; SAC, Standardized Assessment of Concussion[19]; NP Battery, neuropsychological test battery.

MTBI subjects impaired on neuropsychological testing seven days post-MTBI, however, must be balanced against the false-positive rate of 9 percent identified in the normal control group.

Based on these findings, the combination of brief screening instruments appropriate for emergent use in the evaluation of MTBI it was recommended, with more extensive neuropsychological testing recommended to assess recovery further out from injury. Recent research on measuring neuropsychological recovery is reviewed further in chapter 10.

Conclusion

In summary, recent findings from prospective MTBI studies, in both sports and the general MTBI population, allow us to draw several conclusions about the acute cognitive effects and early recovery of cognitive functioning after MTBI:

- There are measurable impairments in cognitive functioning after MTBI, without LOC, PTA, or focal neurologic deficits.
- There are signs of measurable improvement in cognitive functioning as early as within minutes to hours after MTBI.
- Much like the symptom profile, cognitive functioning follows a gradual course of complete recovery in the first week in most cases.

- Memory is the most susceptible to change after MTBI but also shows a complete recovery within days.
- Gross disorientation and other frank cognitive abnormalities are less common in MTBI.
- Prospective empirical findings also illustrate a significant overlap between symptom and cognitive recovery during the first several days following MTBI.

10

Neuropsychological Recovery

The topic of long-term cognitive recovery after MTBI not only has garnered the most attention from clinicians and researchers over the past decade but also has generated the overwhelming majority of clinical studies. For many reasons, it makes sense that neuropsychologists have been at the forefront of this movement and made an unparalleled contribution to advancing the science of MTBI. First, MTBI, more than any other clinical entity, is by its very nature a *neuropsychological* construct. That is, the scientific evidence clearly indicates the pathophysiology of MTBI as a neurologic injury, but clinical studies also clearly illustrate the influence of psychological factors in predicting long-term outcome after MTBI. Based on their understanding of both neurologic and psychological principles, it could be argued that neuropsychologists are uniquely suited to wear both hats in researching and clinically managing MTBI.

This review of neuropsychological recovery after MTBI benefits from the combined work of several respected MTBI researchers more than a decade ago and a number of superb meta-analytic studies that in the last three years have provided an exhaustive summary of the literature on this topic. Here I provide a brief historical summary of some of the earlier work, and then more extensively summarize several recent meta-analyses on the cognitive effects of MTBI and sport-related concussion.

Foundational Neuropsychological Studies

The work of Dikmen and colleagues significantly advanced the neuropsychological understanding of TBI, and in particular MTBI, more than a decade ago. This group published a series of studies on neuropsychological and neurobehavioral outcome in a large group of TBI patients, a portion of whom were classified as MTBI. In 1995, Dikmen et al.[25] published a study on neuropsychological outcome at one year postinjury in 436 adult TBI patients and 121 general trauma control participants; the clinical sample included 161 MTBI patients. It should be noted that inclusion criteria for this study required a head injury serious enough to require a hospitalization, thereby building a possible selection bias for the MTBI population (i.e., including only the most severe end of the MTBI category).

Their results showed that TBI was associated with neuropsychological impairments at one year postinjury but, more important, that the magnitude and pervasiveness of impairments in cognitive functioning were highly dependent on TBI severity. In other words, their findings were the first to indicate a "dose–response" relationship between TBI severity and neuropsychological outcome.[26] Specifically, there was a significant dose–response relationship between length of coma (period of unconsciousness defined by time to follow commands) and level of cognitive impairment one year postinjury.

With respect to MTBI patients (defined by time to follow commands < 1 hr postconcussion), however, neuropsychological performance was comparable to trauma controls, with no significant differences between these two groups in spite of large sample sizes and use of a comprehensive battery of neuropsychological measures. These findings were considered consistent with other controlled studies of MTBI[27,28] from that era.

Others have pointed out that if we look at the 1995 data from Dikmen et al.[25] and expand the threshold for MTBI from 1 hr time to follow commands to 1–24 hr time, there is still essentially no difference between trauma controls and MTBI subjects on a lengthy neuropsychological test battery.[26] Selective impairments on measures of attention and memory start to emerge as the severity of head injury increases, particularly when time to follow commands exceeds 24 hr. Dikmen et al. concluded that although the neuropsychological and psychosocial sequelae following MTBI, natural history of recovery from MTBI, and causes of persistent sequelae or complicated recoveries were of great interest and debate for many years, their results were consistent with prior prospective, control studies indicating that MTBI (e.g., GCS score of 13–15 or time to follow commands < 1 hr) in general was not associated with long-term persistent neuropsychological impairments. They added that this finding was evident in spite of inclusion of patients with potential structural lesions or secondary complications that were serious enough to require hospitalization without inclusion of the milder of the MTBI spectrum.

Larrabee[26] summarized the impact of MTBI on neuropsychological functioning as effect sizes from the Dikmen et al. study, and two quasi-prospective studies.[29,30] Also included was the effect size from a fourth study[31] that selected MTBI patients on the basis of persisting complaints. Effect sizes from the Dikmen et al.,[25] Alterman et al.,[29] and Bornstein et al.[30] studies were quite small;[25,30] in fact, the Alterman et al. effect size (−0.21) was actually in the negative direction, with MTBI patients performing *better* than non-MTBI controls. The effect size from the Leininger et al. study[31] (0.57) is much larger than the prospective or quasi-prospective studies but, again, is based on MTBI patients selected on the basis of continuing complaints, which likely creates a significant selection bias confounding the study.

Larrabee[26] also compared these published MTBI effect sizes to those from groups with financial incentives in head trauma (0.47)[14] and chronic pain (0.48),[32] concluding that meta-analytic data from well-conducted studies showed good long-term neuropsychological recovery for most persons after MTBI.

The Meta-Analytic Age

In 1997, Binder, Rohling, and Larrabee[33] published a meta-analytic review of neuropsychological studies of MTBI. Studies were included as long as patients were studied at least three months after MTBI, patients were selected because of a history of MTBI rather than on the basis of persistent complaints, and the study's attrition rate was less than 50 percent for longitudinal studies. The meta-analyses were restricted to studies of adult MTBI, and no studies of children were included. In total, eight published papers with 11 samples that met the meta-analysis criteria were included. Sample sizes from the eight studies ranged from 18 to 282 MTBI patients. Across the 11 study samples, 314 MTBI patients and 308 controls were available for analyses. Using a more liberal D statistic for effect size, after weighting for sample size, the mean effect size for the 11 samples was 0.12 (SD = 0.18). This is equivalent to approximately one-eighth of a standard deviation. Comparable computations using the more conservative G statistic were also performed, with a mean effect size of 0.07 (SD = 0.17) after weighting for sample size. These findings and those from other meta-analytic studies can be interpreted according to accepted standards for the magnitude of effects sizes (i.e., 0.2 = small effect size, 0.5 = moderate effect size, 0.8 = large effect size).

Binder et al.[33] also compared these effect sizes to the effect size of financial incentives on symptoms and impairment after MTBI, which was estimated in the order of 0.47,[14] and the neuropsychological effects of hypertension, estimated at 0.67.[34] When looking at the positive predictive value of neuropsychological testing, the authors reported that, when the prevalence of brain injury was 5 percent, the positive predictive value was only 32 percent when both sensitivity and specificity were set at 0.90, but that it was improbable that neuropsychological procedures have sensitivity and specificity values as high as 0.90 when assessing subtle brain dysfunction. Lower sensitivity or specificity also results in lower positive predictive value and increases the negative predictive value. The authors concluded that the average effect of MTBI on neuropsychological performances is undetectable, and that the clinician assessing an MTBI patient is more likely to be correct when diagnosing no brain injury and less likely to be correct when diagnosing.

In a follow-up report, Binder[35] reported on the clinical implications of the earlier meta-analytic review. He concluded that, on a chronic basis, 7–8 percent of MTBI patients remained symptomatic and 14 percent are disabled from work. He also added that the association between MTBI and cognitive deficits, symptoms, and disability may not be causal. That is, empirical data suggest that MTBI patients have more psychosocial problems prior to injury than do noninjured persons. Finally, he concluded that the possibility of a neurologic basis for sustained neuropsychological problems cannot be completely dismissed, but there was very little evidence at the time for neurologic causation of most persisting complaints after MTBI.

Several more recent meta-analytic studies have either replicated or advanced the work of Binder, Larrabee, and others nearly a decade ago. In 2003, Schretlen and Shapiro[36] published a quantitative review of the effects of TBI on cognitive functioning. This report was a unique contribution to the literature by way of its *quantitative* review of cognitive functioning across the spectrum of TBI severity. They conducted a meta-analysis of 39 mostly cross-sectional studies of the cognitive effects of MTBI and moderate-severe TBI from the acute phase through long-term follow-up. These studies reported 48 comparisons of TBI patients ($n = 1,716$) and control subjects ($n = 1,164$). Averaged across all follow-up periods, the effect of moderate-severe TBI (weighted mean Cohen's $d = -0.74$) was more than three times the effect of MTBI (weighted mean $d = -0.24$) on overall cognitive functioning. The natural logarithm of the follow-up interval correlated very strongly with estimates of D among patients with MTBI, but less so among those with moderate-severe TBI. In total, 24 estimates of the impact of MTBI on overall cognitive functioning at various follow-up intervals were computed.

For MTBI, the initial weighted d of -0.41 was moderate and indicated the average MTBI patient tested during the first six days postinjury performed at about the 33rd percentile (i.e., within the average range) of matched controls. By 30–89 days postinjury, the weighted mean pooled d of -0.08 represented a trivial effect and indicates that the average MTBI patient performed at the 48th percentile (i.e., the middle of the average range) of matched controls. More than 89 days postinjury, the MTBI patients marginally outperformed matched controls, with a mean effect size of $+0.04$. Taking a different perspective, only 28 percent of the overall test score distributions produced by MTBI patients during the first six days postinjury and their matched controls do not overlap, and this drops to less than 3 percent by one month postinjury for MTBI patients. Finally, the overall cognitive test performance by MTBI patients was essentially indistinguishable from that of matched controls by one month postinjury.

Schretlen and Shapiro[36] concluded that their meta-analysis provided compelling evidence that overall cognitive recovery after MTBI occurred at an exponential rate, based on the natural logarithms at follow-up intervals correlating strongly (R values of 0.67 and 0.70) with effect sizes. In brief, they summarized their meta-analysis on recovery by stating that overall cognitive functioning recovers most rapidly during the first few weeks following MTBI, and essentially returns to baseline within one to three months.

In 2005, Belanger et al.[37] published a report on factors moderating neuropsychological outcome following MTBI. They conducted a meta-analysis of the relevant literature to determine the impact of MTBI across several cognitive domains (global cognitive functioning, attention, executive functions, fluency, memory acquisition, delayed memory, language, and visual spatial skills). The analyses were based on 39 studies involving 1,463 MTBI patients and 1,191 controls. The overall effect of MTBI on neuropsychological functioning was moderate ($d = 0.54$). However, findings were moderated by cognitive domain, time since injury, patient characteristics, and sampling methods. Acute effects (less than three months postinjury) of MTBI were greatest for delayed memory and fluency ($d = 1.03$ and 0.89, respectively).

In unselected or prospective samples, the overall analysis revealed no residual neuropsychological impairments by three months postinjury ($d = 0.04$). In contrast, clinic-based samples and samples including participants in litigation were associated with greater cognitive sequelae of MTBI ($d = 0.74$ and 0.78, respectively, at three months or greater). Litigation was associated with stable or *worsening* cognitive functioning over time. In the studies using unselected samples by 90 days postinjury, no individual cognitive domain was significantly different from zero, with the exception of fluency, which was an outlier finding based on only one study.

Belanger et al.[37] concluded that MTBI had little to no effect on neuropsychological functioning by three months or more postinjury in an MTBI population, both in global cognitive functioning and in specific cognitive domains. Their data suggested that the time since injury effect reported by Schretlen and Shapiro[36] was also generalizable across most cognitive domains, not just global cognitive functioning. This study also highlighted the point that sampling method (i.e., clinic-based vs. unselected samples) is paramount when studying the neuropsychological outcome after MTBI.

Frencham, Fox, and Maybery[38] also conducted a meta-analytic review of neuropsychological studies of MTBI since 1995. This meta-analysis summarized research that was published since the previous meta-analyses by Binder and colleagues[14,39,40] and included data collected at any stage postinjury. Their meta-analysis revealed 17 studies that were suitable for inclusion, from which effect sizes on neuropsychological effects were aggregated. The overall effect size was $G = 0.32$, where speed of processing had the largest effect ($G = 0.47$). The authors also merged postacute effect sizes with those reported in Binder and colleague's meta-analyses, which yielded a nonsignificant result ($G = 0.11$). Similar to the findings of other researchers, Frencham and colleagues concluded that time since injury was found to be the most significant moderator of neuropsychological outcome after MTBI, with effect sizes approaching zero further out from MTBI.

Iverson[41] took an innovative approach to studying the neuropsychological effects of MTBI by converting effect sizes from previous meta-analytic studies to a standard metric (i.e., that used for IQ scores with a mean of 100 and standard deviation of 15). This exercise illustrated that moderate and severe brain injuries have a pronounced negative effect on cognitive functioning, but MTBIs have essentially no measurable effect on cognitive functioning after the acute recovery period. That is, MTBI subjects one to three months postinjury were found to have essentially normal cognitive functioning. Iverson then compared the overall cognitive effects of MTBI with other conditions based on a quantitative summary of hundreds of studies and thousands of patients. This approach also revealed that the effects of MTBI on overall neuropsychological functioning after the acute recovery period are very small, considerably smaller than the effects of depression, bipolar disorder, ADHD,

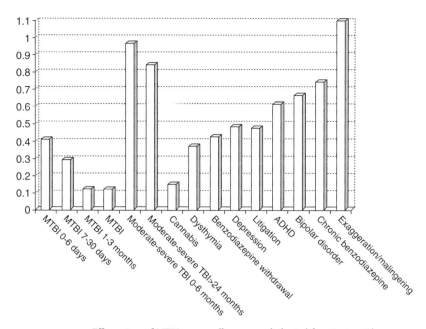

FIGURE 10.1. Effects sizes of MTBI on overall neuropsychological functioning. The overall effect on cognitive or neuropsychological functioning is reported. Effect sizes less that 0.3 should be considered very small and difficult to detect in individual patients because the patient and control groups largely overlap. From Iverson[41] with permission.

benzodiazepine use/withdrawal, litigation, and malingering neuropsychological test performance (Figure 10.1). Similarly, MTBI was discovered to have among the smallest effects on memory functioning in comparison to other conditions such as AIDS/HIV, ADHD, systemic cancer, multiple sclerosis, and schizophrenia (Figure 10.2).

Neuropsychological Recovery After Sport-Related Concussion

In the past five years, several studies of sport-related concussion have also demonstrated a rapid return to normal neuropsychological functioning in the first several days after injury. A review of the literature reflects estimates of symptom and cognitive recovery ranging anywhere from several hours to several weeks after sport-related concussion.[3,42–58] Findings vary based mostly on the methods applied in a respective study.

Pellman et al.[59] evaluated post-MTBI neuropsychological test performance of professional football players studied between 1996 and 2001. Their

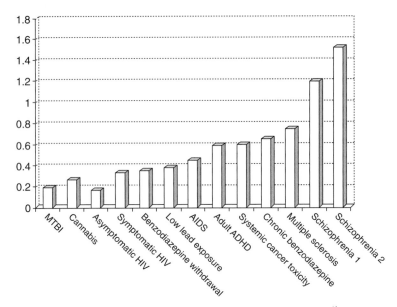

FIGURE 10.2. Effects sizes of MTBI on memory functioning. From Iverson[41] with permission.

findings indicated that professional football players demonstrated generally intact neuropsychological test performance within several days after MTBI relative to preinjury baseline performance levels. There was no evidence of neurocognitive decline even in a subgroup of athletes that were withheld from sport participation for seven or more days. Bleiberg et al.[60] also reported a full recovery in cognitive performance during the first three to seven days after sport-related concussion in boxers.

Few prospective, controlled studies have demonstrated evidence of significant neuropsychological impairment beyond seven days postinjury, and when the case, this impairment extends out only approximately 10–14 days postinjury.[58,61] As in the general MTBI literature, however, neuropsychological effect sizes are very small further out from sport-related concussion. McClincy et al.[62] also reported that subjective symptoms of "feeling slowed down" outlasted impairment on neuropsychological testing, challenging earlier suggestions that impairment on cognitive testing outlasts self-reported concussive symptoms.

Similar to the general MTBI neuropsychological literature, a 2005 meta-analysis by Belanger and Vanderploeg[63] was conducted to determine the impact of sport-related concussion on cognitive functioning. Their analysis was based on 21 studies involving 790 cases of concussion and 2,014 controls. The overall effect of concussion ($d = 0.49$) was quite comparable to the effect sizes sited in those prior meta-analyses in the non-sport-related MTBI population, including that from the earlier meta-analysis by the same researchers,[37] which reported an overall effect size of $d = 0.54$.

Belanger and Vanderploeg reported that acute effects (within 24 hr of injury) of concussion were greatest for delayed memory, memory acquisition, and global cognitive functioning, with effect sizes between 1.0 and 1.42. There were no residual neuropsychological impairments, however, when neuropsychological testing was completed beyond seven days postinjury. The findings from their meta-analysis were moderated by specific cognitive domain in the comparison group utilized (normal control group vs. individual, preinjury baseline as self-control). The authors concluded that their meta-analysis provided compelling evidence that sport-related concussion results in no significant effect on neuropsychological functioning by 7–10 days postinjury in the athletic population at large.

Conclusion

In summary, several meta-analyses and prospective studies over the past decade indicate that uncomplicated MTBI is most often followed by a favorable course of neuropsychological recovery over a period of days to weeks, with no indication of permanent impairment on neuropsychological testing by three months postinjury.

11

Influence of Acute Injury Characteristics on Recovery

Posttraumatic Amnesia and Loss of Consciousness

As noted in part one, there has historically been great emphasis placed on acute injury characteristics in defining and grading the severity of TBI. The assumption that unconsciousness, for example, is an essential characteristic of MTBI has been perpetuated throughout the medical literature over the past several decades. Even today, modern-day medical textbooks still cite unconsciousness as a defining characteristic essential to the diagnosis of concussion or MTBI.

Data from recent studies, however, demonstrate clear and consistent evidence of cerebral dysfunction in cases of concussion without classic indicators of MTBI, such as loss of consciousness (LOC) and posttraumatic amnesia (PTA). These data support a movement in the neurosciences toward a revised definition of concussion that emphasizes an *alteration* (as opposed to a loss) of consciousness or mental status as the hallmark of concussion and stress the potential seriousness of all head injuries, even what has historically been referred to as a simple "bell ringer."[64] Critical care physicians and other health care professionals responsible for the initial identification and diagnosis of MTBI should especially be aware that the diagnosis of concussion does not require an LOC, significant amnesia, or other focal neurologic abnormalities associated with more severe head injury.

In fact, several studies over the past decade indicate that unconsciousness and measurable PTA are relatively uncommon in cases where an alteration in mental status or other defining features of MTBI are clearly evident. Prospective studies have documented that LOC of more than 1–2 min is atypical in MTBI patients with GCS scores between 13 and 15. Furthermore, unconsciousness in the range of 20–30 min or more is rarely observed in the case of MTBI.[65]

With respect to PTA, Paniak et al.[66] generated a normative profile of MTBI in a sample of 119 adults with MTBI, drawn from consecutive admissions to two hospital emergency departments. Their results show that (1) retrograde amnesia (RGA) was not reported or was generally very brief, (2) RGA was not reported unless PTA was also present, and (3) the median ratio of PTA to RGA duration, when both were reported, was 300:1. Similar reports[67] also reference a much higher frequency and longer duration of PTA than RGA following MTBI.

Our body of work in sport-related concussion has documented the relatively infrequency of LOC and amnesia in several large-scale prospective studies. Table 8.1 (page 90) provides a summary of the acute injury characteristics in a case series of 658 sport-related MTBIs from three large prospective studies of high school and collegiate athletes. Again, the advantages that these injuries are all witnessed and evaluated immediately enhances the reliability of documenting the presence and duration of LOC and amnesia.

As reflected in the data, unconsciousness is observed between approximately 7 percent and 18 percent of all sport-related MTBIs and cases in the studies, whereas PTA and RGA are observed between roughly 15 percent and 40 percent of the time. Overall, however, there was no observed unconsciousness or measurable PTA in 67 percent of the 658 cases studied. Furthermore, the median duration of total amnesia in these cases is in the order of 5–10 min, with rare instances of amnesia persisting beyond 30 min. Additionally, unconsciousness not only was an infrequent occurrence but also had a very short median duration in the order of 5 sec. There were no instances of unconsciousness greater than 5 min in this case series of 658 MTBIs.

The relative importance of LOC and amnesia in predicting outcome has been debated for many years. For both LOC and amnesia, the discussion divides into three main questions.[68] First, are either or both of these acute injury characteristics reliable indicators of brain injury severity, suggesting a deeper cerebral lesion or greater magnitude of cerebral dysfunction than in cases without LOC or amnesia? Second, should the presence of LOC or PTA influence the acute management of MTBI? Finally, is either or both of these acute injury characteristics predictive of short- and long-term outcome following MTBI?

The literature consistently indicates evidence that prolonged periods of unconsciousness or amnesia have a significant impact on neuropsychological and functional outcome after more severe forms of TBI. Patients with comas lasting one to two weeks have worse outcomes than patients with coma lasting less than 24 hr.[25] The predictive power of LOC and PTA in more severe forms of TBI has naturally extended to the application of these constructs in studies of MTBI. The more compelling question, however, remains as to whether or not *brief* LOC and PTA are predictive of outcome after MTBI.

It is now commonly considered that brief LOC, as is almost always the case if present at all in MTBI with GCS score of 13–15, is noteworthy but not likely critical. Studies[65,69] have also demonstrated that brief LOC is not predictive of neuropsychological test performance beyond the very acute phase of postinjury, with no appreciable difference in cognitive test performance between MTBI patients with and without LOC at one week postinjury. As summarized by Iverson et al.,[68] researchers studying trauma patients reported that there is no association between *brief* LOC and short-term neuropsychological outcome[31,46,65,69] or vocational outcome.[70] Iverson et al. conclude that LOC is not a reliable predictor of worse short-, medium-, or long-term outcome in trauma patients. Based on recent studies, it is also quite apparent that LOC is also not predictive of outcome following sport-related concussion.[46]

Similarly, while PTA is an important marker of TBI severity, the power of brief PTA in predicting neuropsychological and functional outcome after MTBI is less robust. While PTA may be associated with more severe effects and slower recovery during the acute phase,[46,57,58,71,72] it is not predictive of subacute or long-term outcome. Other reports have supported clinical lore that RGA may indicate a more severe grade of brain injury than that manifested by PTA, which may also extend recovery time. Collins et al.[72] reported that athletes with RGA and PTA were significantly more likely to have poor neuropsychological test performance and symptom recovery two days postinjury than those without amnesia, but there was no difference between good and poor presentation groups in terms of on field LOC.

One study[46] distinguished the importance of LOC and amnesia as acute severity indicators but not necessarily predictive of outcome. In this study of 91 sport-related concussions, the severity of neurocognitive abnormalities detected in standardized testing immediately after injury was correlated with both LOC and PTA. Subjects who experienced a brief period of PTA after injury were immediately more impaired than those who did not experience PTA, and subjects who had sustained observed LOC displayed the most severe neurocognitive impairments immediately after MTBI (see Figure 11.1).[68]

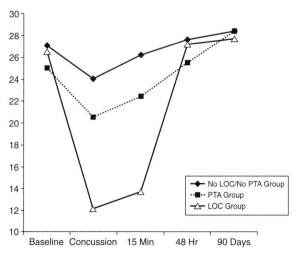

FIGURE 11.1. Cognitive recovery by MTBI subjects with and without LOC and PTA. From McCrea et al.[46] with permission.

Empirical evidence from this perspective study of human subjects supported results from earlier animal research models of MTBI,[73] suggesting that concussive brain injury may occur in the absence of LOC but that more severe grades of cerebral trauma manifest as more observable neurologic dysfunction and neurocognitive impairment.

Findings from this particular study were also informative with respect to the early natural history of neurocognitive abnormalities during the acute phase of MTBI. Injured subjects without PTA or LOC displayed the fastest recovery during the acute phase, without significant cognitive impairments (as a group) by 15 min after injury. Interestingly, subjects who experienced LOC remained more impaired than did subjects without LOC or PTA at 15 min but closed the gap of recovery within two days, such that there were no statistically significant differences between the three clinical groups at 48 hr after injury. Nearly all subjects with or without LOC and PTA demonstrated full recovery in cognitive functioning within two days after injury.

In summary, these findings suggest that brief LOC and PTA may indicate a more severe gradient of MTBI that correlates with cognitive impairment and other MTBI-related deficits during the most acute phase, which is not predictive of eventual cognitive recovery and functional outcome after MTBI. Two important distinctions require attention with respect to the influence of

Mild Traumatic Brain Injury and Postconcussion Syndrome

LOC and amnesia following MTBI. First, brief LOC or amnesia as defined in the accepted parameters to define MTBI are noteworthy, but not likely critical in terms of acute injury management or predicting outcome. Second, more extended periods of LOC and amnesia are perhaps of greater diagnostic and clinical value during the very acute injury phase (within the first 48–72 hr) but do not likely have long-term prognostic significance. When including moderate and more severe forms of TBI, PTA and LOC of longer duration have much more significant diagnostic and prognostic value.[74] Several studies, however, have demonstrated that sociodemographic and other non-injury-related variables have at least equal and perhaps greater significance in predicting outcome after MTBI.[6,75–78]

Complicated Versus Uncomplicated MTBI

There is also continued debate on whether focal trauma reflected on brain neuroimaging (e.g., contusions, hematomas, edema on acute head CT or MRI) is associated with poorer short-, mid-, or long-term outcome after MTBI. Several studies have reported poorer neuropsychological test performance during the acute period (days to weeks) postinjury, as well as poorer outcome one to five years post-MTBI in patients with "complicated" MTBI evidenced by structural injury visualized on neuroimaging. Other studies have reported no differences between those with complicated and uncomplicated MTBI.

A study by Iverson[79] investigated the effects of complicated versus un-complicated MTBI on acute neuropsychological outcome. All MTBI patients underwent CT scanning on the day of injury and completed a small battery of neuropsychological tests within the first two weeks of injury. Iverson sorted the MTBI patients into two groups on the basis of having normal (uncomplicated MTBI) or abnormal (complicated MTBI) CT scan during the acute phase. In-jured patients were then matched to normal controls on the basis of age, education, gender, and nature of injury (e.g., motor vehicle accident, fall, as-sault). In total, 100 MTBI patients were studied, 50 in each group.

Iverson's results showed that patients with complicated MTBIs performed significantly more poorly on some of the neuropsychological tests, but the effect sizes were small to medium, and the two groups could not be differ-entiated using logistic regression analysis. McCauley et al.[80] reported that complicated MTBI was not associated with increased risk for PCS at three months postinjury. Iverson et al.[81] have also demonstrated that patients with uncomplicated MTBI could not be reliably differentiated from patients with substance abuse problems on measures of concentration, memory, and processing speed.

Overall, complicated MTBI characterized by structural brain damage visualized on acute neuroimaging may increase the risk for slow or incomplete recovery after MTBI but is not perfectly predictive of good or poor outcome in the majority of MTBI patients.[68]

12

Measuring Neurophysiologic Recovery

Advances in functional neuroimaging not only provide valuable insights on the mechanisms underlying the pathophysiology of MTBI but also may provide a new platform for measuring the early course of neurophysiologic recovery following TBI. For many reasons, functional magnetic resonance imaging (fMRI) may have various technological, methodological, and practical advantages over other functional imaging platforms when it comes to studying recovery and the effects of rehabilitation in TBI. Several investigators have implemented fMRI in the study of MTBI, including recent studies that have applied fMRI techniques in the investigation of sport-related concussion.[82,83]

Our research group lead by Thomas Hammeke and others at the Medical College of Wisconsin has included fMRI studies as part of a larger project tracking recovery of cognitive functioning, postconcussive symptoms, and postural stability in athletes following concussion. In keeping with the traditional sports concussion research model, all subjects undergo preseason baseline testing on several concussion assessment measures of cognitive functioning, symptoms, and postural stability. These measures are then repeated at several time points postinjury to track recovery after MTBI. Matched control subjects also complete identical protocol to establish the normal pattern of performance on serial testing.

As part of our local study, all subjects with AAN grade 2 or grade 3 concussions (symptoms persisting beyond 15 min, with evidence of PTA or LOC) undergo fMRI studies the day following injury (typically within 15 hr of injury) and approximately 45 days postinjury. Noninjured control subjects matched to the injured player on the basis of age, educational level, and preseason cognitive test performance also undergo fMRI studies.

A Sternberg task is used as an activation paradigm to assess memory-scanning speed under conditions of different memory load. In the Sternberg task, a string of two, four, or six digits is visually presented to the subject for 2 sec. Following a delay of a few seconds, a probe digit is visually displayed to the subject, and he is instructed to manually indicate whether the probe digit was part of the previously presented string of digits. An event-related design is used so that the hemodynamic response to each set size could be studied. The event-related design also allows an analysis of set size effects during the encoding (digits at presentation), maintenance (digit rehearsal during the delay), and retrieval (probe digit presentation and response) phases of the Sternberg task.

With respect to the behavioral fMRI data, findings from our fMRI study indicate that concussed players are less accurate than their matched controls in performing the Sternberg task on the day following injury. Concussed players had a generally slower reaction time across all set sizes on day 1 postinjury that resolved by six weeks postinjury. Furthermore, this deficit was most robust in players with the most severe gradient of concussion characterized by documented unconsciousness associated with their concussion.

When looking at the functional imaging data, our noninjured control subjects showed a pattern of cortical and subcortical activation increases in response to the Sternberg task, most of which is explained by relationship to memory load (set size) of the task. Regions showing increased activation with increasing memory load included the supplementary motor area (SMA), pre-SMA and anterior cingulate, bilateral basal ganglia (putamen and caudate), left premotor region, and biparietal zones that are often activated in verbal working memory tasks. The memory load effect was most apparent in the encoding phase and maintenance phase of the task, and not in the response phase.

Our preliminary analyses of the MTBI subjects activation profiles show that, on the day following injury, the hemodynamic response is diminished relative to the controls in the select brain regions (e.g., the SMA/pre-SMA and anterior cingulate) during the encode phase of the task. The diminished activation is not accounted for by task accuracy or deficits on neurocognitive tests but is negatively correlated with reaction time. Furthermore, the effect of diminished activation is almost entirely accounted for by those subjects who had LOC associated with their concussion. Interestingly, there are no activation differences in any regions of interest between the injured and control subjects by six weeks postinjury.

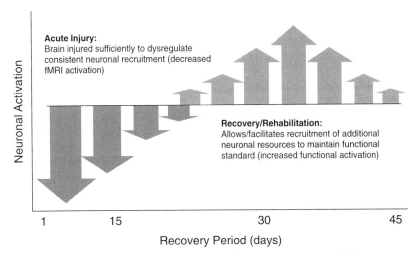

FIGURE 12.1. Neurophysiologic recovery after MTBI: functional model of MTBI effects and recovery measuring chlinically meaningful cerebral change. For moderate/severe TBI, the model gives implications for amplitude/course/reversibility.

In summary, these preliminary data suggest that MTBI subjects show an abnormal profile of cerebral activation in response to cognitive demands during the most acute period following MTBI, which is characterized by decreased activation of select neuronal circuits in the frontal lobes. Furthermore, this effect is most evident in MTBI subjects who had LOC associated with their concussion, perhaps suggesting a more severe gradient of injury marked by LOC, similar to findings from clinical studies.[46] At six weeks postinjury, there are no cerebral activation deficits in the injured subjects, suggesting full neurophysiologic recovery relative to the acute phase.

When considered in the context of other f MRI studies of MTBI, these data provide the basis for a theoretical model of neurophysiologic recovery after MTBI (see Figure 12.1). That is, during the most acute period (within 24 hr postinjury), there is decreased cerebral activation on f MRI studies, suggesting an inability for the brain to recruit additional neuronal resources to meet environmental cognitive demands when the brain is in its most severe state of neurometabolic disarray. Other studies during the subacute recovery phase (e.g., 30 days postinjury) indicate a pattern of increased activation, with the hypothesis that the brain is recruiting additional neuronal resources to meet cognitive demands. The final study point in our investigation (45 days postinjury) indicates that the brain has returned to a normal neurophysiologic state, consistent with parallel findings of complete clinical recovery of symptoms, cognitive functioning, and all other functional deficits.

Conclusion

In summary, preliminary findings from prospective studies utilizing fMRI illustrate the neurophysiologic effects of MTBI during the most acute phase that correspond with acute symptoms and cognitive dysfunction. The course of neurophysiologic recovery also appears to correlate with the demonstrated natural course of symptom and cognitive recovery after MTBI as the brain returns to a normal physiologic state within weeks of injury.

13

■ ■ ■

Functional Outcome After MTBI

MTBI: A Different Animal

As noted in part one, the total cost and societal impact of TBI are substantial. In more severe forms of TBI, the resulting impact on the patient's academic, vocational, social, and overall independent functioning can be devastating. In moderate and severe TBI, acute injury severity (measured by LOC, PTA, GCS, etc.) is the single strongest predictor of functional outcome.

And therein lies the great divide in TBI. While injury severity is indeed the strongest predictor of recovery and outcome in the case of moderate and severe TBI, this principle does not apply below a certain threshold. GCS score, duration of unconsciousness, and length of PTA have been the most commonly studied criteria linked to prognosis after moderate and severe TBI, while other innovative approaches have investigated the predictive power of time to follow commands and other acute injury characteristics. The classic work of Dikmen and colleagues[25,84] has been incredibly informative in identifying factors that predict neuropsychological, neurobehavioral, and functional outcome after moderate and severe TBI.

Unfortunately, acute injury characteristics have not been as effective in predicting outcome following milder forms of TBI. When we look at the MTBI population, for example, injury-related factors (e.g., unconsciousness, amnesia) have not empirically been the most powerful predictors of which patients are at greatest risk of poor functional outcome or persistent PCS. Rather, non-injury-related factors such as premorbid psychosocial issues, postinjury stressors, alcohol and drug problems, and litigation factors are more commonly predictive of the potential for poor outcome after MTBI.

The complexity of this dilemma has not only stumped researchers investigating MTBI outcome, but also drastically overhauled head injury management in most hospital emergency departments. The highest priority for emergency department physicians and staff is now to rule out neurosurgical emergency associated with TBI, as it should be. Beyond that, however, emergency medical personnel now realize that full assessment of the noninjury factors associated with MTBI outcome is beyond their means and expertise, so the MTBI patient is most often medically cleared and released from the emergency department immediately after the head CT is negative. In some instances, but not all, patients are instructed to follow up with their primary care physicians to address any persistent symptoms after MTBI. Quite often, however, MTBI patients are completely lost from any medical follow-up.[64]

A 2000 study by Ponsford et al.[76] indicated that a range of factors, other than those directly reflecting the severity of injury (LOC and PTA), appear to be associated with outcome following MTBI. Factors associated with persistent symptoms at three months post-MTBI included a history of previous neurologic or psychiatric problems, being a student, and presence of other life stressors. The subgroup of MTBI patients who were still suffering symptoms at three months were highly distressed, and their lives were still significantly disrupted. This group of patients, however, did not have a more severe gradient of injury than those who followed a complete recovery in the same time frame, based on acute injury characteristics. This study again underscores the importance of preexisting personality traits, psychological needs, and psychosocial stress as factors that influence outcome after MTBI, likely above and beyond the influence of specific acute injury characteristics under a certain threshold.

Measuring Outcome After MTBI

Iverson et al.[68] provided an extensive summary of the literature on return to work after MTBI. MTBI patients have consistently higher return work rates than those with moderate to severe TBI,[85–90] but not all individuals return to work at the same rate after MTBI. When isolating the MTBI sample, it appears that those with less severe MTBI (GCS of 15, no LOC) have higher return-to-work rates than those with more severe grades of MTBI (e.g., GCS of 13–14 and positive LOC). Iverson points out that there is substantial variability in return-to-work rates after MTBI, which are stratified based on time since injury. Overall, the highest percentage of MTBI subjects returned to work at some point after injury, and the percentage increased over the course of recovery further out from injury. Iverson highlights a number of methodological differences across studies that likely contribute to this variability in return-to-work rates, including differences in definitions of posted return to work, varied MTBI inclusion criteria, and variations in preinjury work status.

Another important component of functional outcome after MTBI relates to psychological and psychosocial functioning. Several studies have identified a higher risk of depression and anxiety after MTBI, much like in the case of chronic pain and other medical conditions. Depression is purportedly common following TBI at any severity level, with varied prevalence rates.

In 2006, Meares et al.[91] investigated the association between PCS and neuropsychological and psychological outcome in 122 general trauma patients, many of whom also had orthopedic injuries, around five days following MTBI. Individuals with PCS reported significantly more psychological symptoms, and large effect sizes were present on the psychological measures, so the difference between participants with PCS was greater on psychological than on neuropsychological measures. Their analyses also revealed a relationship between opiate analgesia and depression, anxiety and stress, and opioids and reduced learning. In summary, the authors concluded that psychological factors are present much earlier than previously considered in the development of PCS.

Iverson et al.[68] summarize the results from several studies on depression prevalence rates in MTBI. Across seven studies between 1996 and 2005, the rate of depression in MTBI ranged from roughly 12 percent to 44 percent of MTBI subjects. Iverson[92] also highlights the possible confound of misdiagnoses of persistent PCS in patients with depression, due to significant overlap in the symptom criteria for each diagnosis.

A summary statement on the prognosis for MTBI from the WHO Collaborating Centre Task Force on Mild Traumatic Brain Injury was published in 2004 and was one of a series of papers from the WHO task force.[1] With relevance to prognosis and outcome, the committee concluded that adults with MTBI frequently experienced early cognitive deficits and postconcussive symptoms (most commonly headache) in the early weeks after injury, but insufficient attention has been paid to the role of psychological distress or pain from associated injuries and the etiology of these symptoms. The committee went on to add that most adults follow a good recovery course after MTBI, and that a host of non-injury-related factors are important to consider when symptoms and disability persist after MTBI.

Conclusion

Overall, functional recovery after MTBI follows a course similar to that of symptom and neuropsychological recovery. That is, the overwhelming majority of MTBI patients return to normal independent functioning, social functioning, and work in their normal capacity within a period of days to weeks after injury. Also, similar to the studies on cognitive and symptoms recovery, non-injury-related factors often play a significant role in functional outcome. That is, MTBI subjects with preexisting medical or psychological problems, high levels of psychosocial stress at time of injury, and poor social support systems after injury are potentially at risk of poorer functional outcome associated with MTBI.

14

■ ■ ■

Exceptions to the Rule:
Potential Long-Term Effects of MTBI

In addition to the methodological advantages of the sports concussion research model outlined in part one, the sports setting also provides other circumstances unique from the typical, general MTBI population. Specifically, sports are perhaps the only setting in which people are highly motivated to return to the very activity that caused their initial injuries immediately after experiencing an MTBI. This scenario in turn creates a situation in which the athlete is exposed to risk of repeat MTBI, in some cases involving multiple head injuries over a relative short period of time (e.g., days, weeks, or months within the same sport season).

Rare Catastrophic Outcome

Extremely rare instances of death or severe, permanent disability have been reported in association with "second impact syndrome" (or delayed cerebral edema).[93–95] In brief, second impact syndrome is hypothesized as a catastrophic outcome following recurrent MTBI in which a second injury occurs before an athlete completes a full recovery from a first injury and while the brain remains in a state of vulnerability to more severe effects from additional trauma. Documented case studies indicate a course of rapid deterioration after a second injury, typically while an athlete remains symptomatic within days of their initial injury. In many instances, the athlete collapses and a course characterized by coma and respiratory failure ensues as a result of increased intracranial pressure from severe vascular congestion and brainstem herniation. The end result is often death or permanent disability. This occurrence is extremely rare even in a sports setting, and the vascular/physiologic mechanisms underlying second impact syndrome remain under debate.

Effects of Recurrent MTBI

More common than second impact syndrome is the occurrence of exposure to repeat sport-related concussion without catastrophic outcome, which still raises concerns about cumulative or long-term effects of recurrent MTBI. Several studies of sport-related concussion have investigated two important questions focused on potential long-term consequences of MTBI. First, can exposure to repetitive subconcussive blows result in chronic neuropsychological impairments or other problems? For example, there has been debate about whether heading exposure in soccer may lead to chronic brain injury, characterized by neurocognitive deficits and persistent postconcussive symptomatology. Several recent studies of soccer and football, however, have demonstrated that participation in these sports and heading exposure does not result in chronic neuropsychological impairment or other problems.[96,97]

A second question relates to whether there are any cumulative effects of recurrent concussion. Previous studies[98] have reported a stepwise increase in risk for subsequent concussion based on the number of prior concussions in a players history. While there is no definitive answer as to "how many is too many?" it appears that individuals with a history of three or more concussions may be at potentially at increased risk for recurrent concussion, lengthier recovery time after concussion, and potentially even long-term risks later in life.

In a study of 4,251 college football players, Guskiewicz et al.[98] reported a significant association between reported number of previous concussions and likelihood of incident concussion during the study period (see Table 14.1). Players reporting a history of three or more previous concussions were three times more likely to suffer a concussion than players with no prior history of concussion. Slowed recovery time was also associated with a history of multiple previous concussions, as 30 percent of those with three or more previous concussions had symptoms lasting more than one week, compared with just 14.6 percent of those with one previous concussion (see Table 14.2). This study also demonstrated that the greatest risk of repeat concussion is during the acute recovery phase within the first 7–10 days after a concussion, suggesting that the brain remains in a state of cerebral vulnerability to repeat trauma during the early recovery period.

Table 14.1 Association Between Concussion History and Risk of Incident Concussion

NO. PREVIOUS CONCUSSIONS	INCIDENT CONCUSSIONS*	ATHLETE SEASONS	ESTIMATED ATHLETE-EXPOSURES	RATE (95% CI) PER 1,000 ATHLETE-EXPOSURES	RATE RATIO (95% CI)	MULTIVARIATE ADJUSTED RATE RATIO (95% CI)
0	122 (3.7%)	3,265	185,060	0.66 (0.54, 0.78)	1.0 (referent)	1.0 (referent)
1	41 (5.4%)	756	42,850	0.96 (0.66, 1.25)	1.5 (1.0, 2.1)	1.4 (1.0, 2.1)
2	15 (10.5%)	143	8,105	1.85 (0.91, 2.79)	2.8 (1.6, 4.8)	2.5 (1.5, 4.1)
3+	10 (12.7%)	79	4,478	2.23 (0.85, 3.62)	3.4 (1.8, 6.5)	3.0 (1.6, 5.6)

*Number (percentage) of players from each concussion group (chi squared = 30.11, df = 3, $p < .001$).
From Guskiewicz et al.[98] with permission.

In 2004, Iverson et al.[99] examined the association between history of multiple concussions and cumulative effects on symptoms and cognitive functioning. At baseline, athletes with a history of multiple concussions reported more symptoms than did athletes with no history of concussion, but there was no difference in their cognitive test performance. Approximately two days after concussion, athletes with a prior history of concussion also performed significantly lower on memory testing than did athletes with a single concussion.

In 2005, however, Iverson et al.[100] reported that there was no measurable effect of one or two previous concussions on baseline neuropsychological test performance or symptom reporting in 867 high school and college athletes. They concluded that if there is a cumulative effect of one or two previous concussions, it is very small and essentially undetectable with current methods. Collie et al.[101] also concluded that there is no relationship between the number of previous self-reported episodes of concussion and current neurocognitive functioning.

Potential Long-Term Risks

Finally, questions have been raised as to whether MTBI may increase the risk of lifetime incidence of depression, eventual cognitive decline, or dementia. TBI has been identified as a potential risk factor for the occurrence (or early expression) of neurodegenerative dementing disorders, including Alzheimer's disease (AD) and Parkinson's syndrome, and other psychiatric disorders such as clinical depression.[102–112]

At least one study has suggested that the severity of head injury is related to the magnitude of AD risk and that the risk of AD associated with head injury involving LOC was approximately double that associated with head injury without LOC.[113] In that same study, however, even head injury without LOC significantly increased the risk of AD relative to no head injury history at all. It has been suggested that head injury is a risk factor for AD and that this risk is heightened among carriers of the e4 allele of the apolipoprotein E gene (APOE e4). This generalization, however, appears to have greater relevance to moderate and severe TBI than it does in MTBI.

Guskiewicz et al.[102] investigated the association between previous head injury and the likelihood of developing mild cognitive impairment (MCI) and AD in a unique group of retired professional football players with previous head injury exposure. Questionnaire data were obtained from 2,552 retired

Table 14.2 Length of MTBI Recovery by Concussion History

NO. PREVIOUS CONCUSSIONS*	RAPID RECOVERY (SYMPTOMS < 1 DAY)	GRADUAL RECOVERY (SYMPTOMS 1–7 DAYS)	PROLONGED RECOVERY (SYMPTOMS >7 DAYS)
0 ($n = 122$)	37 (30.3%)	76 (62.3%)	9 (7.4%)
1 ($n = 41$)	16 (39.0%)	19 (46.3%)	6 (14.6%)
2 ($n = 15$)	5 (33.3%)	7 (46.7%)	3 (20.0%)
3+ ($n = 10$)	0 (0%)	7 (70.0%)	3 (30.0%)

Data are expressed as No. (%) of players with concussion. *Fisher's exact test ($p = .03$). From Guskiewicz et al.[98] with permission.

professional football players that collected information on their health history, history of previous concussion, and other demographic variables. A second questionnaire focusing on memory and issues related to MCI was then completed by a subset of 758 retired professional football players (and a spouse or immediate caregiver), and results on MCI were then cross-tabulated with the results from the original health questionnaire subset of retired athletes. Sixty-one percent of the sample reported sustaining at least one concussion during their professional football career, and 24 percent sustained three or more previous concussions. There was a significant association between recurrent concussion and clinically diagnosed MCI and self-reported memory impairments. Retired players with three or more reported concussion had a fivefold prevalence of MCI diagnosis and a threefold prevalence of reported significant memory problems compared with subjects who had no prior history of concussion (see Figure 14.1). Although there was no association between recurrent concussion and AD, the researchers observed an earlier onset of AD in retirees than in the general American male population.

Guskiewicz et al.[102] concluded that the onset of dementia-related syndromes may be initiated by repetitive cerebral concussions in professional football players. A similar study by Guskiewicz and colleagues currently in press also suggests that a history of repetitive concussion may increase the risk of lifetime incidence of depression.[115]

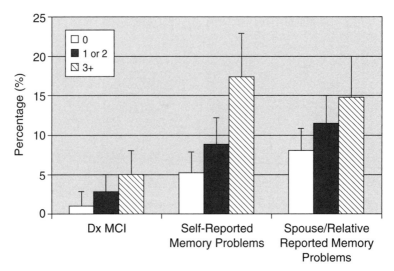

FIGURE 14.1. Association between concussion history, late-life memory problems, and mild cognitive impairment (MCI). Figures represent percentage of retired professional football players 50 or more years of age with a diagnosis of MCI and memory problems (self-reported and reported by a spouse or close relative) by concussion history (none, one, two, and three or more). Error bars indicate 95% confidence intervals ($p < .007$). From Guskiewicz et al.[98] with permission.

Conclusion

Preliminary studies suggest that, while a single, uncomplicated MTBI is a transient neurologic event followed by relatively rapid and spontaneous recovery, recurrent MTBI may be associated with longer recovery time and persistent symptoms, as well as potentially increasing the lifetime risk of psychiatric and neurologic problems. Further study on this issue is required, and prospective, longitudinal studies of athletes can provide a sound methodology to do so.

Part Three Top 10 Conclusions

1. MTBI symptoms gradually resolve over a period of days to weeks in the overwhelming majority of cases.

2. Measurable impairments in cognitive functioning are evident during the acute phase following MTBI, in the

absence of unconsciousness, amnesia, or focal neurologic deficits.

3. MTBI is most often followed by a favorable course of cognitive recovery over a period of days to week, with no indication of permanent impairment on neuropsychological testing by three months postinjury.

4. Preliminary findings illustrate neurophysiologic effects of MTBI that follow a course of recovery consistent with the natural course of symptom and cognitive recovery as the brain returns to a normal physiologic state within days to weeks of injury.

5. Acute injury characteristics (e.g., unconsciousness, amnesia) are noteworthy in diagnosing and grading the severity of TBI, but brief unconsciousness and amnesia are not predictive of recovery and outcome after MTBI.

6. Complicated MTBI characterized by structural injury visualized on acute neuroimaging may increase the risk of slow or incomplete recovery after MTBI but is not perfectly predictive of outcome in the majority of MTBI patients.

7. The overwhelming majority of MTBI patients follow a favorable course of functional recovery by returning to normal occupational, social, and independent functioning within days to weeks after injury.

8. Overall, the natural history of MTBI in children and adults is characterized by gradual, full recovery in symptoms, cognition, and general functioning within several days to weeks of injury, and the true incidence of persistent symptoms or impairments that negatively affect the patient's general functioning is very low.

9. In uncomplicated MTBI, persistent symptoms and poor functional outcome are often associated with non-injury-related variables, including demographic, psychosocial, medical, motivational, and other situational factors.

10. Preliminary data suggest that recurrent MTBI may be associated with longer recovery time and may increase the long-term risk of psychiatric and neurologic problems.

References

1. Carroll LJ, Cassidy JD, Peloso PM, et al. Prognosis for mild traumatic brain injury: results of the WHO Collaborating Centre Task Force on Mild Traumatic Brain Injury. *J Rehabil Med* 2004:84–105.

2. Garraway M, Macleod D. Epidemiology of rugby football injuries. *Lancet* 1995;345:1485–87.

3. Macciocchi SN, Barth JT, Alves W, Rimel RW, Jane JA. Neuropsychological functioning and recovery after mild head injury in collegiate athletes. *Neurosurgery* 1996;39:510–14.

4. McCrory PR, Ariens T, Berkovic SF. The nature and duration of acute concussive symptoms in Australian football. *Clin J Sport Med* 2000;10:235–38.

5. Riemann BL, Guskiewicz KM. Effects of mild head injury on postural stability as measured through clinical balance testing. *J Athl Train* 2002;35:19–25.

6. Bazarian JJ, Wong T, Harris M, Leahey N, Mookerjee S, Dombovy M. Epidemiology and predictors of post-concussive syndrome after minor head injury in an emergency population. *Brain Inj* 1999;13:173–89.

7. Paniak C, Reynolds S, Phillips K, Toller-Lobe G, Melnyk A, Nagy J. Patient complaints within 1 month of mild traumatic brain injury: a controlled study. *Arch Clin Neuropsychol* 2002;17:319–34.

8. Lowdon IM, Briggs M, Cockin J. Post-concussional symptoms following minor head injury. *Injury* 1989;20:193–94.

9. Paniak C, Phillips K, Toller-Lobe G, Durand A, Nagy J. Sensitivity of three recent questionnaires to mild traumatic brain injury-related effects. *J Head Trauma Rehabil* 1999;14:211–19.

10. Cline DM, Whitley TW. Observation of head trauma patients at home: a prospective study of compliance in the rural south. *Ann Emerg Med* 1988;17:127–31.

11. Lidvall HF, Linderoth B, Norlin B. Causes of the post-concussional syndrome. *Acta Neurol Scand Suppl* 1974;56:3–144.

12. Lidvall HF, Linderoth B, Norlin B. Causes of the post-concussional syndrome: IX. Psychological tests. *Acta Neurol Scand* 1974;50:64–71.

13. Landre N, Poppe CJ, Davis N, Schmaus B, Hobbs SE. Cognitive functioning and postconcussive symptoms in trauma patients with and without mild TBI. *Arch Clin Neuropsychol* 2006;21:255–73.

14. Binder LM, Rohling ML. Money matters: a meta-analytic review of the effects of financial incentives on recovery after closed-head injury. *Am J Psychiatry* 1996;153:7–10.

15. Paniak C, Reynolds S, Toller-Lobe G, Melnyk A, Nagy J, Schmidt D. A longitudinal study of the relationship between financial compensation and symptoms after treated mild traumatic brain injury. *J Clin Exp Neuropsychol* 2002;24:187–93.

16. Paniak C, Toller-Lobe G, Melnyk A, Nagy J. Prediction of vocational status three to four months after treated mild traumatic brain injury. *J Musculoske Pain* 2000;8:193–200.

17. Lovell MR, Collins MW. Neuropsychological assessment of the college football player. *J Head Trauma Rehabil* 1998;13:9–26.

18. Alexander MP. Mild traumatic brain injury: pathophysiology, natural history, and clinical management. *Neurology* 1995;45:1253–60.

19. McCrea M, Randolph C, Kelly JP. *Standardized Assessment of Concussion (SAC): Manual for Administration, Scoring and Interpretation*, 2nd ed. Waukesha, WI: CNS Inc., 2000.

20. Kelly JP, Rosenberg JH. Diagnosis and management of concussion in sports. *Neurology* 1997;48:575–80.

21. McCrea M, Guskiewicz KM, Marshall SW, et al. Acute effects and recovery time following concussion in collegiate football players: the NCAA Concussion Study. *JAMA* 2003;290:2556–63.

22. Barr WB, McCrea M. Sensitivity and specificity of standardized neurocognitive testing immediately following sports concussion. *J Int Neuropsychol Soc* 2001;7:693–702.

23. Giza CC, Hovda DA. The neurometabolic cascade of concussion. *J Athl Train* 2001;36:228–235.

24. McCrea M, Barr WB, Guskiewicz K, et al. Standard regression-based methods for measuring recovery after sport-related concussion. *J Int Neuropsychol Soc* 2005;11:58–69.

25. Dikmen S, Machamer J, Winn HR, Temkin N. Neuropsychological outcome at one-year post head injury. *Neuropsychology* 1995;9:80–90.

26. Larrabee GJ. Neuropsychological outcome, post concussion symptoms, and forensic considerations in mild closed head trauma. *Semin Clin Neuropsychiatry* 1997;2:196–206.

27. Dikmen S, McLean A, Temkin N. Neuropsychological and psychosocial consequences of minor head injury. *J Neurol Neurosurg Psychiatry* 1986;49:1227–32.

28. Levin HS, Mattis S, Ruff RM, et al. Neurobehavioral outcome following minor head injury: a three-center study. *J Neurosurg* 1987;66:234–43.

29. Alterman AI, Goldstein G, Shelly C, Bober B, Tarter RE. The impact of mild head injury on neuropsychological capacity in chronic alcoholics. *Int J Neurosci* 1985;28:155–62.

30. Bornstein RA, Podraza AM, Para MF, et al. Effect of minor head injury on neuropsychological performance in asympotmatic HIV-1 infection. *Neuropsychology* 1993;7:228–34.

31. Leininger BE, Gramling SE, Farrell AD, Kreutzer JS, Peck EA III. Neuropsychological deficits in symptomatic minor head injury patients after concussion and mild concussion. *J Neurol Neurosurg Psychiatry* 1990;53:293–96.

32. Rohling ML, Binder LM, Langhinrichsen-Rohling J. Money matters: a meta-analytic review of the association between financial compensation and the experience and treatment of chronic pain. *Health Psychol* 1995;14:537–47.

33. Binder LM, Rohling ML, Larrabee GJ. A review of mild head trauma. Part I: meta-analytic review of neuropsychological studies. *J Clin Exp Neuropsychol* 1997;19:421–31.

34. Waldstein SR, Manuch SB, Ryan CM, Muldoon MF. Neuropsychological correlates of hypertension: review and methodologic considerations. *Psychol Bull* 1991;110:451–468.

35. Binder LM. A review of mild head trauma. Part II: clinical implications. *J Clin Exp Neuropsychol* 1997;19:432–57.

36. Schretlen DJ, Shapiro AM. A quantitative review of the effects of traumatic brain injury on cognitive functioning. *Int Rev Psychiatry* 2003;15:341–49.

37. Belanger HG, Curtiss G, Demery JA, Lebowitz BK, Vanderploeg RD. Factors moderating neuropsychological outcomes following mild traumatic brain injury: a meta-analysis. *J Int Neuropsychol Soc* 2005;11:215–27.

38. Frencham KA, Fox AM, Maybery MT. Neuropsychological studies of mild traumatic brain injury: a meta-analytic review of research since 1995. *J Clin Exp Neuropsychol* 2005;27:334–51.

39. Binder LM, Rohling ML, Larrabee GJ. A review of mild head trauma. Part I: meta-analytic review of neuropsychological studies. *J Clin Exp Neuropsychol* 1997;19:421–31.

40. Binder LM. A review of mild head trauma. Part II: clinical implications. *J Clin Exp Neuropsychol* 1997;19:432–57.

41. Iverson GL. Outcome from mild traumatic brain injury. *Curr Opin Psychiatry* 2005;18:301–17.

42. McCrea M, Kelly JP, Randolph C, et al. Standardized assessment of concussion (SAC): on-site mental status evaluation of the athlete. *J Head Trauma Rehabil* 1998;13:27–35.

43. Collins MW, Grindel SH, Lovell MR, et al. Relationship between concussion and neuropsychological performance in college football players. *JAMA* 1999;282:964–70.

44. Echemendia RJ, Putukian M, Mackin RS, Julian L, Shoss N. Neuropsychological test performance prior to and following sports-related mild traumatic brain injury. *Clin J Sport Med* 2001;11:23–31.

45. McCrea M. Standardized mental status testing on the sideline after sport-related concussion. *J Athl Train* 2001;36:274–79.

46. McCrea M, Kelly JP, Randolph C, Cisler R, Berger L. Immediate neurocognitive effects of concussion. *Neurosurgery* 2002;50:1032–42.

47. Erlanger D, Kaushik T, Cantu R, et al. Symptom-based assessment of the severity of a concussion. *J Neurosurg* 2003;98:477–84.

48. Cremona-Meteyard SL, Geffen GM. Persistent visuospatial attention deficits following mild head injury in Australian Rules football players. *Neuropsychologia* 1994;32:649–62.

49. Maddocks DL, Dicker GD, Saling MM. The assessment of orientation following concussion in athletes. *Clin J Sport Med* 1995;5:32–35.

50. Maddocks D, Saling M. Neuropsychological deficits following concussion. *Brain Inj* 1996;10:99–103.

51. McCrory PR, Bladin PF, Berkovic SF. Retrospective study of concussive convulsions in elite Australian rules and rugby league footballers: phenomenology, aetiology, and outcome. *BMJ* 1997;314:171–74.

52. Hinton-Bayre AD, Geffen GM, Geffen LB, McFarland KA, Friis P. Concussion in contact sports: reliable change indices of impairment and recovery. *J Clin Exp Neuropsychol* 1999;21:70–86.

53. Macciocchi SN, Barth JT, Littlefield L, Cantu RC. Multiple concussions and neuropsychological functioning in collegiate football players. *J Athl Train* 2001;36:303–6.

54. McCrea M. Standardized mental status assessment of sports concussion. *Clin J Sport Med* 2001;11:176–81.

55. Warden DL, Bleiberg J, Cameron KL, et al. Persistent prolongation of simple reaction time in sports concussion. *Neurology* 2001;57:524–26.

56. Hinton-Bayre AD, Geffen G. Severity of sports-related concussion and neuropsychological test performance. *Neurology* 2002;59:1068–70.

57. Collins MW, Field M, Lovell MR, et al. Relationship between postconcussion headache and neuropsychological test performance in high school athletes. *Am J Sports Med* 2003;31:168–73.

58. Lovell MR, Collins MW, Iverson GL, et al. Recovery from mild concussion in high school athletes. *J Neurosurg* 2003;98:296–301.

59. Pellman EJ, Lovell MR, Viano DC, Casson IR, Tucker AM. Concussion in professional football: neuropsychological testing—part 6. *Neurosurgery* 2004;55:1290–305.

60. Bleiberg J, Cernich AN, Cameron K, et al. Duration of cognitive impairment after sports concussion. *Neurosurgery* 2004;54:1073–80.

61. McClincy MP, Lovell MR, Pardini J, Collins MW, Spore MK. Recovery from sports concussion in high school and collegiate athletes. *Brain Inj* 2006;20:33–39.

62. McClincy MP, Pardini J, Lovell M, Fazio V, Collins M. Relationship Between Symptom Report of Feeling Slowed Down and Cognitive Performance on Neuropsychological Testing. Poster presented at the

34th Annual Meeting of the International Neuropsychological Society; St. Louis, MO; 2005.

63. Belanger HG, Vanderploeg RD. The neuropsychological impact of sports-related concussion: a meta-analysis. *J Int Neuropsychol Soc* 2005;11:345–57.

64. Bazarian JJ, Blyth B, Cimpello L. Bench to bedside: evidence for brain injury after concussion—looking beyond the computed tomography scan. *Acad Emerg Med* 2006;13:199–214.

65. Iverson GL, Lovell MR, Smith SS. Does brief loss of consciousness affect cognitive functioning after mild head injury? *Arch Clin Neuropsychol* 2000;15:643–48.

66. Paniak C, MacDonald J, Toller-Lobe G, Durand A, Nagy J. A preliminary normative profile of mild traumatic brain injury diagnostic criteria. *J Clin Exp Neuropsychol* 1998;20:852–55.

67. Cantu RC. Posttraumatic retrograde and anterograde amnesia: pathophysiology and implications in grading and safe return to play. *J Athl Train* 2001;36:244–48.

68. Iverson GL, Lange RT, Gaetz M, Zasler ND. Mild TBI. In: Zasler ND, Katz DI, Zafonte RD, eds. *Brain Injury Medicine: Principles and Practice*. New York: Demos Medical Publishing, 2006:333–71.

69. Lovell MR, Iverson GL, Collins MW, McKeag D, Maroon JC. Does loss of consciousness predict neuropsychological decrements after concussion? *Clin J Sport Med* 1999;9:193–98.

70. Hanlon RE, Demery JA, Martinovich Z, Kelly JP. Effects of acute injury characteristics on neuropsychological status and vocational outcome following mild traumatic brain injury. *Brain Inj* 1999;13: 873–87.

71. Pellman EJ, Viano DC, Casson IR, Arfken C, Powell J. Concussion in professional football: injuries involving 7 or more days out—part 5. *Neurosurgery* 2004;55:1100–19.

72. Collins MW, Iverson GL, Lovell MR, McKeag DB, Norwig J, Maroon J. On-field predictors of neuropsychological and symptom deficit following sports-related concussion. *Clin J Sport Med* 2003;13:222–29.

73. Ommaya AK, Gennarelli TA. Cerebral concussion and traumatic unconsciousness. Correlation of experimental and clinical observations of blunt head injuries. *Brain* 1974;97:633–54.

74. van der Naalt J, van Zomeren AH, Sluiter WJ, Minderhoud JM. One year outcome in mild to moderate head injury: the predictive value of acute injury characteristics related to complaints and return to work. *J Neurol Neurosurg Psychiatry* 1999;66:207–13.

75. Nolin P. Executive memory dysfunctions following mild traumatic brain injury. *J Head Trauma Rehabil* 2006;21:68–75.

76. Ponsford J, Willmott C, Rothwell A, et al. Factors influencing outcome following mild traumatic brain injury in adults. *J Int Neuropsychol Soc* 2000;6:568–79.

77. Bazarian J, Hartman M, Delahunta E. Minor head injury: predicting follow-up after discharge from the Emergency Department. *Brain Inj* 2000;14:285–94.

78. Luis CA, Vanderploeg RD, Curtiss G. Predictors of postconcussion symptom complex in community dwelling male veterans. *J Int Neuropsychol Soc* 2003;9:1001–15.

79. Iverson G. Predicting slow recovery from sport-related concussion: the new simple-complex distinction. *Clin J Sport Med* 2007;17:31–37.

80. McCauley SR, Boake C, Levin HS, Contant CF, Song JX. Postconcussional disorder following mild to moderate traumatic brain injury: anxiety, depression, and social support as risk factors and comorbidities. *J Clin Exp Neuropsychol* 2001;23:792–808.

81. Iverson GL, Lange RT, Franzen MD. Effects of mild traumatic brain injury cannot be differentiated from substance abuse. *Brain Inj* 2005;19:11–18.

82. Jantzen KJ, Anderson B, Steinberg FL, Kelso JA. A prospective functional MR imaging study of mild traumatic brain injury in college football players. *Am J Neuroradiol* 2004;25:738–45.

83. Chen JK, Johnston KM, Frey S, Petrides M, Worsley K, Ptito A. Functional abnormalities in symptomatic concussed athletes: an f MRI study. *Neuroimage* 2004;22:68–82.

84. Haltiner AM, Temkin NR, Winn HR, Dikmen SS. The impact of posttraumatic seizures on 1-year neuropsychological and psychosocial outcome of head injury. *J Int Neuropsychol Soc* 1996;2:494–504.

85. Stambrook M, Moore AD, Peters LC, Deviaene C, Hawryluk GA. Effects of mild, moderate and severe closed head injury on long-term vocational status. *Brain Inj* 1990;4:183–90.

86. Dikmen SS, Temkin NR, Machamer JE, Holubkov AL, Fraser RT, Winn HR. Employment following traumatic head injuries. *Arch Neurol* 1994;51:177–86.

87. Asikainen I, Kaste M, Sarna S. Patients with traumatic brain injury referred to a rehabilitation and re-employment programme: social and professional outcome for 508 Finnish patients 5 or more years after injury. *Brain Inj* 1996;10:883–99.

88. Dawson DR, Levine B, Schwartz ML, Stuss DT. Acute predictors of real-world outcomes following traumatic brain injury: a prospective study. *Brain Inj* 2004;18:221–38.

89. Hawley CA, Ward AB, Magnay AR, Mychalkiw W. Return to school after brain injury. *Arch Dis Child* 2004;89:136–42.

90. Uzzell BP, Langfitt TW, Dolinskas CA. Influence of injury severity on quality of survival after head injury. *Surg Neurol* 1987;27:419–29.

91. Meares S, Shores EA, Batchelor J, et al. The relationship of psychological and cognitive factors and opioids in the development of the postconcussion syndrome in general trauma patients with mild traumatic brain injury. *J Int Neuropsychol Soc* 2006;12:792–801.

92. Iverson GL. Misdiagnosis of the persistent postconcussion syndrome in patients with depression. *Arch Clin Neuropsychol* 2006;21:303–10.

93. Cantu RC. Second-impact syndrome. *Clin Sports Med* 1998;17:37–44.

94. Kelly JP, Nichols JS, Filley CM, Lillehei KO, Rubinstein D, Kleinschmidt-DeMasters BK. Concussion in sports. Guidelines for the prevention of catastrophic outcome. *JAMA* 1991;266:2867–69.

95. Saunders RL, Harbaugh RE. The second impact in catastrophic contact-sports head trauma. *JAMA* 1984;252:538–39.

96. Guskiewicz KM. No evidence of impaired neurocognitive performance in collegiate soccer players. *Am J Sports Med* 2002;30:630.

97. Straume-Naesheim TM, Andersen TE, Dvorak J, Bahr R. Effects of heading exposure and previous concussions on neuropsychological performance among Norwegian elite footballers. *Br J Sports Med* 2005;39(suppl 1):i70–i77.

98. Guskiewicz KM, McCrea M, Marshall SW, et al. Cumulative effects associated with recurrent concussion in collegiate football players: the NCAA Concussion Study. *JAMA* 2003;290:2549–55.

99. Iverson GL, Gaetz M, Lovell MR, Collins MW. Cumulative effects of concussion in amateur athletes. *Brain Inj* 2004;18:433–43.

100. Iverson GL, Brooks BL, Lovell MR, Collins MW. No cumulative effects for one or two previous concussions. *Br J Sports Med* 2006;40:72–75.

101. Collie A, McCrory P, Makdissi M. Does history of concussion affect current cognitive status? *Br J Sports Med* 2006;40:550–51.

102. Guskiewicz KM, Marshall SW, Bailes J, et al. Association between recurrent concussion and late-life cognitive impairment in retired professional football players. *Neurosurgery* 2005;57:719–26.

103. Graves AB, White E, Koepsell TD, et al. The association between head trauma and Alzheimer's disease. *Am J Epidemiol* 1990;131:491–501.

104. Holsinger T, Steffens DC, Phillips C, et al. Head injury in early adulthood and the lifetime risk of depression. *Arch Gen Psychiatry* 2002;59:17–22.

105. Mayeux R, Ottman R, Tang MX, et al. Genetic susceptibility and head injury as risk factors for Alzheimer's disease among community-dwelling elderly persons and their first-degree relatives. *Ann Neurol* 1993;33:494–501.

106. Mortimer JA, French LR, Hutton JT, Schuman LM. Head injury as a risk factor for Alzheimer's disease. *Neurology* 1985;35:264–67.

107. O'Meara ES, Kukull WA, Sheppard L, et al. Head injury and risk of Alzheimer's disease by apolipoprotein E genotype. *Am J Epidemiol* 1997;146:373–84.

108. Rasmusson DX, Brandt J, Martin DB, Folstein MF. Head injury as a risk factor in Alzheimer's disease. *Brain Inj* 1995;9:213–19.

109. Schofield PW, Tang M, Marder K, et al. Alzheimer's disease after remote head injury: an incidence study. *J Neurol Neurosurg Psychiatry* 1997;62:119–24.

110. Shalat SL, Seltzer B, Pidcock C, Baker EL, Jr. Risk factors for Alzheimer's disease: a case-control study. *Neurology* 1987;37:1630–33.

111. The Canadian Study of Health and Aging: risk factors for Alzheimer's disease in Canada. *Neurology* 1994;44:2073–80.

112. van Duijn CM, Tanja TA, Haaxma R, et al. Head trauma and the risk of Alzheimer's disease. *Am J Epidemiol* 1992;135:775–82.

113. Guo Z, Cupples LA, Kurz A, et al. Head injury and the risk of AD in the MIRAGE study. *Neurology* 2000;54:1316–23.

114. Guskiewicz KM, Ross SE, Marshall, SW. Postural stability and neuropsychological deficits after concussion in collegiate athletes. *J Athl Training* 2001;36:263–273.

115. Guskiewicz KM, Marshall SW, Bailes J, McCrea M, Harding H, Matthews A, Register Mihalik J, Cantu RC. *Recurrent concussion and risk of depression in retired professional football players.* In press. Med Sci Sport Exer.

PART FOUR

IMPLICATIONS FOR RETHINKING POSTCONCUSSION SYNDROME

In parts one through three, the scientific literature on the epidemiology, acute effects, natural history, and outcome associated with mild traumatic brain injury (MTBI) have been summarized. There is no question that MTBI is a highly prevalent form of injury that has substantial economic and societal impact. Scientific advances over the past decade have also demonstrated a rather clear pathophysiology of MTBI, now commonly known as the "neurometabolic cascade," that leaves the brain in a state of neurophysiologic disarray during the acute phase after injury.

There has also been a convergence between findings from basic science and clinical studies of the natural history of acute effects and recovery following MTBI. Prospective, controlled studies demonstrate a pattern of clinical recovery in symptoms, cognitive functioning, and other functional parameters over a period of several days in an overwhelming majority of MTBI cases that closely parallels findings on the course of neurophysiologic recovery. Functional neuroimaging studies have also now extended our knowledge of physiologic recovery from animal studies to humans, which also demonstrate the brain's return to normal neurophysiologic functioning within days to weeks after MTBI. In sum, there is solid scientific evidence demonstrating the neuropathophysiologic basis for MTBI as a transient process followed by spontaneous recovery typically over the course of several days to weeks postinjury.

As promised at the outset of this text, our ultimate aim is to transfer the latest science of MTBI to clinical applications that guide clinicians to an evidence-based approach to assessment and treatment that will ultimately enhance outcome and reduce disability associated with MTBI. Part four turns to the construct of postconcussion syndrome (PCS) and, more specifically, those cases that fall into the category of *persistent* PCS.

PCS is without question one of the most controversial concepts in the neurosciences and has been the subject of healthy debate for decades.[1] The debate typically centers around whether persistent symptoms and other functional impairments that fall outside the expected recover pattern after MTBI are due to neurologic, psychological, or other non-injury-related factors. For years, a lack of scientific evidence has prevented a sound empirical conclusion regarding this dilemma. Furthermore, attempts to address this issue often focused solely on the point of outcome, way late in the game, without considering the entire breadth and depth of scientific evidence on the true natural history of acute and subacute MTBI.

Building on the totality of scientific evidence on the true natural history of MTBI as a foundation, part four highlights the resulting implications that prompt the need to reframe our theoretical and clinical understanding of PCS, which also drives a new approach to the diagnosis and treatment of this disorder. A progressive discussion of issues associated with the definition and epidemiology of PCS will ensue, and theoretical models of PCS are briefly reviewed, along with a new, empirically based perspective of PCS as a *neuropsychological* disorder. Finally, part four discusses practical, evidence-based interventional models intended to improve outcome and reduce persistent disability associated with MTBI.

15

∎∎∎

Defining Postconcussion Syndrome

This discussion of the definition of PCS closely mirrors that in part one on the challenges of defining MTBI itself. Commonly sited definitions and diagnostic criteria for PCS have been criticized for being either too lenient (i.e., inclusive) or too restrictive (i.e., exclusive). Furthermore, the diagnosis of PCS is based exclusively on self-reported signs and symptoms, which several studies have demonstrated to be highly nonspecific to PCS and common to numerous other medical and psychological conditions. So, those problems discussed in part one that complicate our interpretation of the underlying etiology, natural history, and outcome associated with MTBI are also confronted when we address the subset of MTBI patients who are eventually categorized as exhibiting PCS.

PCS Diagnostic Criteria

The two most commonly cited systems for defining and diagnosing PCS come from the 10th edition of the *International Classification of Diseases*[2] (*ICD-10*) and the 4th edition of the *Diagnostic and Statistical Manual of Mental Disorders*[3] (*DSM-IV*). Obviously, both sets of criteria cite the occurrence of head injury as the principal prerequisite for the eventual diagnosis of PCS.

ICD-10 diagnostic criteria for 310.2 postconcussional syndrome (PCS) represent a 1992 revision of criteria that had been in clinical use for more than 20 years (see Box 15.1).[2] According to the *ICD-10* clinical description, the syndrome occurs after head trauma and is characterized by symptoms in three or more categories that are present no later than four weeks postinjury. Interestingly, the *ICD-10* classification system requires a history of head trauma "with a loss of consciousness" to support the diagnosis of PCS. Based on what we now know about the acute injury characteristics of MTBI, this requirement

BOX 15.1 *ICD-10* Diagnostic Criteria for Postconcussional Syndrome

A. History of head trauma with loss of consciousness precedes symptoms onset by maximum of four weeks
B. Symptoms in three or more of the following symptom categories:
- Headache, dizziness, malaise, fatigue, noise tolerance
- Irritability, depression, anxiety, emotional lability
- Subjective concentration, memory, or intellectual difficulties without neuropsychological evidence of marked impairment
- Insomnia
- Reduced alcohol tolerance
- Preoccupation with above symptoms and fear of brain damage with hypochondriacal concern and adoption of sick role

From *International Statistical Classification of Diseases and Related Health Problems*, 10th ed.[2]

would preclude approximately 90 percent of patients from meeting the eventual diagnostic criteria for PCS because no loss of consciousness (LOC) or witnessed unresponsiveness was associated with their injury.

The *ICD-10* criteria for PCS are divided into six separate categories: (1) headache, dizziness, malaise, fatigue, noise intolerance; (2) irritability, depression, anxiety, emotional lability; (3) subjective concentration, memory, or intellectual difficulties without neuropsychological evidence of marked impairment; (4) insomnia; (5) reduced alcohol tolerance; (6) preoccupation with above symptoms and fear of brain damage with hypochondriacal concern and adoption of sick role.

The *DSM-IV* criteria for postconcussional disorder (PCD)[3] require a history of head trauma that has caused significant cerebral concussion (e.g., with LOC, posttraumatic amnesia, or seizures) (see Box 15.2). Again, the reference to the LOC requirement would, based on the latest findings on the acute injury characteristics of MTBI, exclude essentially 90 percent of patients from eligibility for the eventual diagnosis of PCD because there was no LOC associated

BOX 15.2 *DSM-IV* Research Criteria for Postconcussional Disorder

A. A history of head trauma that has caused significant cerebral concussion. Note: The manifestations of concussion include loss of consciousness, posttraumatic amnesia, and, less, commonly, posttraumatic onset of seizures. The specific method of defining this criterion needs to be established by further research.

B. Evidence from neuropsychological testing or quantified cognitive assessment of difficulty in attention (concentrating, shifting focus of attention, performing simultaneous cognitive tasks) or memory (learning or recall of information).

C. Three (or more) of the following occur shortly after the trauma and last at least three months:
   1. Becoming fatigued easily
   2. Disordered sleep
   3. Headache
   4. Vertigo or dizziness
   5. Irritability or aggression on little or no provocation
   6. Anxiety, depression, or affective instability
   7. Changes in personality (e.g., social or sexual inappropriateness)
   8. Apathy or lack of spontaneity

C. The symptoms in criteria B and C have their onset following head trauma or else represent a substantial worsening of preexisting symptoms.

D. The disturbance causes significant impairment in social or occupational functioning and represents a significant decline from a previous level of functioning. In school-age children, the impairment may be manifested by a significant worsening in school or academic performance dating from the trauma.

E. The symptoms do not meet criteria for Dementia Due to Head Trauma and are not better accounted for by another mental disorder (e.g., Amnestic Disorder Due to Head Trauma, Personality Change Due to Head Trauma).

From the *Diagnostic and Statistical Manual of Mental Disorders*, 4th ed.[3]

with their injury. The *DSM-IV* criteria, in contrast to the *ICD-10* system, require "neuropsychological evidence of difficulty in attention or memory."

Additionally, the *DSM-IV* system requires three or more symptoms that last at least three months and have an onset shortly after head trauma or represent substantial worsening of previous symptoms. The *DSM-IV* criteria also require that this disturbance cause significant impairment in social or occupational functioning and represent a significant decline from the patient's previous level of functioning.

Several important points related to the *ICD-10* and *DSM-IV* criteria warrant further discussion.[1] First, these criteria are subjective in nature, even to the extent that there are self-reported cognitive problems but no evidence of impairment on objective neuropsychological testing when it comes to the cognitive symptom category. Additionally, all of the criteria listed are highly nonspecific to MTBI and commonly encountered in a whole host of other medical and psychological conditions. Lastly, the general complexion of these criteria clearly suggests the potential for a psychological or emotional basis for the subjective symptoms of PCS.

Reliability and Validity of PCS Criteria

Several recent studies have evaluated the reliability and clinical utility of the *DSM-IV* and *ICD-10* diagnostic criteria for PCS. Boake et al.[4] compared diagnoses of PCS between the *ICD-10* and the *DSM-IV* classification systems. They studied 178 adults with mild-to-moderate TBI based on a structured interview at three months postinjury. Their results showed that, despite concordance of *DSM-IV* and *ICD-10* symptom criteria ($\kappa = 0.73$), agreement between overall *DSM-IV* and *ICD-10* diagnoses was slight ($\kappa = 0.13$) because few patients met the *DSM-IV* cognitive deficit and clinical significant criteria.

The investigators concluded that agreement between *DSM-IV* PCD and *ICD-10* PCS is limited by different prevalences and thresholds. They also pointed out important implications for clinical and research uses of PCS diagnosis. Specifically, clinicians using the PCS diagnosis must select from alternative criteria sets that may lead to diagnostic decisions that are inconsistent and even incompatible. Future studies that compare the available criteria sets in terms of interrater reliability, specificity, and prognostic value were recommended.

Boake et al.[5] then evaluated the prevalence and specificity of diagnostic criteria for PCS in 178 adults with mild-to-moderate TBI and 104 patients with extracranial trauma. *DSM-IV* and *ICD-10* criteria for PCS were evaluated three months after injury. The results show that prevalence of PCS was higher using *ICD-10* (64 percent) than *DSM-IV* criteria (11 percent). Specificity to TBI was limited because PCS criteria were often fulfilled by patients with extracranial trauma. While 64 percent of TBI patients met the *ICD-10* criteria for PCS, so too did 40 percent of the extracranial trauma sample. Similarly, 7 percent of extracranial trauma patients met the *DSM-IV* criteria for PCS, compared to 11 percent in the TBI sample. Comparing the TBI and extra-cranial samples on each criterion and for *DSM-IV* diagnosis of PCS, a significant odds ratio was observed only for postconcussional symptoms, but there was no difference in the percentages of each sample meeting the cognitive deficit and clinical significance criteria.

Boake et al.[5] concluded that complaints of postconcussional symptoms are not sufficient to make the diagnosis of MTBI. They also pointed out that these findings support the criticism of the World Health Organization (WHO) Collaborating Centre Task Force on Mild Traumatic Brain Injury[6] that, in diagnosing PCS, linking residual symptoms to TBI is a major problem. Boake et al. added that refinement of the PCS diagnostic criteria of *DSM-IV* and *ICD-10* is needed before the criteria can be recommended for routine clinical or research use.

McCauley et al.[7] investigated differences in outcome based on *DSM-IV* diagnoses of PCD versus *ICD-10* criteria for PCS. A series of 319 patients with MTBI and 21 patients with moderate TBI was assessed at three months postinjury with a brief neuropsychological battery and measures of specific outcome domains. Patients with PCD were compared with those without PCD and those with PCS were compared with those without PCS.

There was no substantial pattern of differences between *DSM-IV* and *ICD-10* in the outcome domains of psychiatric symptoms and disorders, social and community integration, health-related quality of life, or global outcomes as measured by the Extended Glasgow Outcome Scale. In spite of significant differences between the two diagnostic criteria sets and different incidence rates for PCD/PCS, outcome in all measured domains was very similar at three months postinjury. They concluded that there is no compelling evidence, based on these outcome domains, to suggest which of the two diagnostic criteria sets is clinically preferred.

Another study investigated the utility of the *ICD-10* diagnostic criteria for PCS symptoms by comparing symptom endorsement rates in a group of patients with MTBI to those of a noninjured control group at one month and three months postinjury.[8] The 110 MTBI patients and 118 control participants were group matched on age, gender, and education level.

Seven of the nine self-reported *ICD-10* PCS symptoms differentiated the groups at one month postinjury, and two symptoms differentiated the groups at three months postinjury. Symptom endorsement rates were higher in the MTBI group at both time periods. Fatiguing quickly and dizziness/vertigo best differentiated the groups at both time periods, while depression and anxiety/tension failed to differentiate the groups at either time period. Collectively, the *ICD-10* PCS symptoms accurately classified the MTBI patients at one month postinjury, with the optimal positive test threshold of endorsement of five symptoms coinciding with a sensitivity and specificity of 73 percent and 61 percent, respectively. The investigators concluded that the *ICD-10* PCS symptoms were unable to accurately classify the MTBI patients at three months postinjury.

Conclusion

In summary, symptom-based diagnosis of PCS is plagued by several difficulties, most notably poor reliability of diagnostic criteria and nonspecificity of PCS symptoms, which are discussed further in chapter 16. Applied studies have failed to demonstrate an edge for either the *ICD-10* or *DSM-IV* for clinical or research use, as both are fraught with similar limitations in reliability and validity.

16

Nonspecificity of Postconcussion Syndrome Symptoms

There is now a substantial empirical literature base showing that PCS symptom report is influenced by factors other than head injury, suggesting that symptoms typically associated with PCS are not specific to head injury. Numerous studies have reported that PCS symptoms are quite common among individuals with various medical or psychological disorders. Others have documented relatively high base rates of postconcussion symptoms in the healthy, normal population.

PCS Symptoms Outside of MTBI

Table 16.1 compares the frequency of endorsement of five common PCS symptoms (headache, dizziness, irritability, memory problems, poor concentration) by MTBI patients and four other non-TBI population samples.[9–13]

Gunstad and Suhr[14] asked 82 undergraduates to report the symptoms they currently experience and then to report the symptoms they would expect to experience if they had suffered either a head injury, orthopedic injury, posttraumatic stress, or depression. No current differences in overall symptoms or in symptom subscales emerged. Their results showed that individuals portraying head injury, posttraumatic stress, and depression expected an increase in total symptoms, though individuals portraying an orthopedic injury did not expect such an increase. Additionally, simulators of head injury, posttraumatic stress, and depression expected equivalent rates of overall symptoms, memory/cognitive complaints, somatic concerns, and distractor symptoms, though head-injured individuals reported fewer affective symptoms than those portraying psychological disorders. Based on their findings, the authors concluded that individuals have a relative lack of specificity in

Table 16.1 Frequency of Common PCS Symptoms in Non-MTBI Samples

	HEADACHE	DIZZINESS	IRRITABILITY	MEMORY PROBLEMS	CONCENTRATION PROBLEMS
College students[9]	36%	18%	36%	17%	42%
Chronic pain[10]	80%	67%	49%	33%	63%
Depressed[11]	37%	20%	52%	25%	54%
PI claimants (non-TBI)[12]	77%	41%	63%	46%	71%
MTBI[13]	42%	26%	28%	36%	25%

Data are expressed as No. (%) of players with concussion. *Fisher's exact test ($p = .03$).
From Guskiewicz et al.[98]

symptom expectation for various disorders, with the implication that symptom checklists for PCS may not be useful for diagnosis.

Wang et al.[15] examined postconcussion-like symptoms in a group of 124 university students and explored their relationships to neuropsychological functioning. Their findings demonstrated that the base rate of postconcussion-like symptoms in a group of healthy university students is relatively high (with at least five symptoms endorsed by more than 45 percent of the total sample) and that postconcussion symptoms were not related to neuropsychological functioning in this normal healthy population.

Iverson and Lange[16] similarly investigated the prevalence of postconcussion-like symptoms in a sample of healthy individuals in a sample of 104 healthy individuals who completed the Short-Form British Columbia Postconcussion Symptom Inventory (BCP-SI), a test designed to measure both the frequency and intensity of *ICD-10* criteria for PCS. The Beck Depression Inventory was also administered to the group. Specific endorsement rates of postconcussion-like symptoms range from 36 percent to 76 percent for any experience of symptoms in the past two weeks, and from 2.9 percent to 15.5 percent for the experience of more severe symptoms. Postconcussion symptoms showed a moderately high correlation with self-reported symptoms of depression. The authors concluded that their findings illustrate that postconcussion-like symptoms are not unique to mild head injury but are commonly found in healthy individuals and highly correlated with depressive symptoms.

Iverson[17] followed up this earlier work with a study examining the prevalence of postconcussion-like symptoms in patients with depression. A total of 64 physician-diagnosed inpatients or outpatients with depression completed the BCP-SI to assess their frequency and severity of PCS symptoms based on *ICD-10* criteria. Specific endorsement of PCS-like symptoms ranged from 31 percent to 86 percent for symptoms rated mild or greater, and from 11 percent to 58 percent for symptoms rated moderate to severe. Approximately 90 percent of patients with depression met liberal self-report criteria for PCS and more than 50 percent met conservative criteria for the diagnosis of PCS.

Lees-Haley et al.[18] compared the rates of PCS symptoms at the time of injury for MTBI claimants ($n = 24$) and claimants reporting other forms of injury ($n = 66$). On checklists surveying their complaints immediately after their injury, MTBI and other injury claimants reported similar levels of many PCS symptoms, including the experience of being dazed, confused, dizzy, and disoriented and having trouble concentrating, numbness or loss of sensation, and loss of memory for some of what happened. The authors concluded that classical PCS complaints experienced immediately after an injury are so non-specific that they have little diagnostic specificity.

Suhr and Gunstad[19] explored whether any subset of self-reported post-concussion symptoms or specific PCS symptom is sensitive and/or specific to head injury in non-self-selected samples with head injury and depression ($n = 32$), head injury without depression ($n = 31$), depression without head injury ($n = 25$), and normal controls ($n = 50$). All subjects completed a self-report PCS symptom scale based on their current symptoms. Their results showed that depression, not head injury status, largely accounted for elevation in PCS symptom reports, including cognitive symptoms. The investigators concluded that report of cognitive PCS symptoms is not specific to head injury and addressed concerns about using symptoms alone to screen for head injury in a general population.

Iverson et al.[1] provide a detailed review of the nonspecificity of ICD-10 and *DSM-IV* diagnostic criteria, including presentation of data on the prevalence of these diagnostic criteria in healthy adults and in patients with depression or fibromyalgia. The authors point out that the general nonspecificity of these criteria potentially leads a clinician to misdiagnose a person with PCS. From their unique data set, Iverson and colleagues have demonstrated that patients with fibromyalgia who report problems with depression, chronic pain, or both are very likely to be misdiagnosed with PCS. Ninety percent of patients with depression or fibromyalgia reported symptoms that can meet diagnostic criteria for PCS based on *ICD-10* criteria. The authors concluded that a person with depression but no history of traumatic brain injury whatsoever is 90 percent likely to meet the *ICD-10* criteria for PCS.

Conclusion

Overall, several studies have demonstrated relatively high rates of PCS symptoms in various samples—from patients with chronic pain, depression, or fibromyalgia, to personal injury claimants and even normal, healthy individuals. Much like the pattern discussed in part three showing that cognitive dysfunction and memory problems after MTBI are often significantly influenced by non-injury-related factors, symptoms that make up the core criteria for the formal diagnosis of PCS are also highly nonspecific to either MTBI or PCS.

17

■ ■ ■

Epidemiology of Postconcussion Syndrome: Another Denominator Problem

Based on the issues discussed in preceding chapters regarding problems with the definition, diagnosis, and nonspecificity of PCS symptoms, questions are also raised about published reports on the assumed prevalence and epidemiology of PCS. Published literature and clinical lore have long purported that approximately 15–20 percent of MTBI patients go on to report subjective symptoms or other complaints beyond three months postinjury that warrant the label of persistent PCS.

The True Tale of PCS Estimates

In 1995, Alexander[20] stated that "at one year after injury, approximately 15 percent of MTBI patients still have disabling symptoms" as part of his review on this particular topic. This figure has been perpetuated in the literature and throughout clinical circles over the past decade. Closer review of the Alexander article, however, notes that his estimate of 15 percent is based on two original references from Rutherford et al. in 1979[21] and McLean et al. in 1983.[22]

While it is correct that Rutherford et al.[21] reported that 19 of 131 (14.5 percent) patients with mild concussion still had symptoms one year postinjury, closer review of this study tells more of the tale. First, the original sample was 145 consecutive cases of concussion admitted to a hospital in Belfast, but only 131 were available for follow-up at one year (adjusted rate = 13.1 percent). More important, of 19 patients who were still reporting symptoms at one year postinjury, eight were involved in law suits and six were suspected of malingering at six weeks postinjury (including five of those that were involved in law suits). Additionally, 10 of the 19 patients reported at least one new symptom at one year that was not endorsed six weeks postinjury. Looking more closely at the data, 6 of the 19 patients had only one symptom, and 7 of the 19 patients had two symptoms at one year postinjury, which are now known to be lower than the base rate of the normal healthy population response to a postconcussion symptom questionnaire and hardly warrant the diagnosis of a syndrome or disorder. The remaining six subjects endorsed between four and nine symptoms, but there was no grouping of interrelated symptoms either at six weeks or at one year postinjury. Therefore, a truer estimate of anything that would come close to the threshold of a disorder or syndrome in this particular study is closer to 3–5 percent of their sample. Even this figure should be interpreted with caution because there were also no control subjects, orthopedically injured or otherwise, in the study, which we know is extremely important given the nonspecificity of symptoms and the potential for false positives in diagnosing PCS.

Similarly, there are also issues as to how the McLean et al.[22] study has been reported in the literature and applied to estimating the prevalence of PCS after MTBI. First, the TBI sample in that study was composed of a *mixture* of mild ($n = 11$), moderate ($n = 8$), and severe ($n = 1$) TBI patients. Also, TBI patients were compared to controls on neurocognitive testing and PCS symptom checklists at three days and *one month* postinjury, but there were no data collected beyond the one month point. The all-severity TBI sample showed significant neuropsychological difficulties at three days postinjury relative to noninjured controls, but there were no group differences at one month postinjury. TBI patients endorsed higher rates of PCS symptoms three days and one month postinjury, which is perhaps not unreasonable given the severity mix in the TBI sample and the timing of the study's assessment endpoint.

Methodological Issues

Historical reports on the epidemiology of PCS have also been confounded by probable ascertainment bias. That is, MTBI patients who are eventually enrolled in studies of PCS likely represent a select subsample of the larger MTBI population, which drastically affects the denominator when attempting to calculate the true incidence of PCS. As noted above, an estimated 25 percent of MTBI or concussion patients never seek any form of medical treatment after their injury and therefore are never accounted for in the PCS incidence denominator. Additionally, most MTBI patients have neither LOC (perhaps as many as 90 percent of all injuries) nor lengthy posttraumatic amnesia (30–50 percent) associated with their injury, which technically precludes them from the diagnosis of PCS based on *DSM-IV* and *ICD-10* criteria.

Quite often, clinicians simply connect the dots between reported occurrence of possible head injury and the subsequent self-report of a single or multiple symptoms and, in forming the diagnosis of PCS, often erroneously ascribe causality to the temporal relationship between the reported incident and subjective complaints. Research studies on PCS also often accrue only those patients referred to clinics because of persistent complaints, which we know are highly nonspecific. Other reports have been based solely on endorsement of items on a PCS checklist, without any collateral investigation of other factors (e.g., depression, anxiety, chronic pain, psychosocial stress, alcohol and drug abuse) known to also cause these symptoms.

Iverson et al.[1] comment on the nonrepresentative samples that often confound PCS studies. They point out that some studies consider patients to have had persistent problems if they endorsed only a single symptom (e.g., headaches or concentration problems) at one year postinjury, whereas endorsement of multiple symptoms that would warrant consideration of a disorder or syndrome at one year is "extremely rare" (<5 percent of subjects).[23]

Revised Estimates of True Incidence of PCS

Without question, the estimate of 15–20 percent of MTBI patients having persistent PCS or disorder is severely inflated. When we factor in the larger estimates of true MTBI epidemiology, problems with the definition and diagnosis of syndrome versus symptoms, and factors other than MTBI that present with a clinical profile reflective of PCS, the true incidence of PCS would appear to be far less than 5 percent of all MTBI patients.[1,24] Depending on how restrictive the criteria are the diagnosis of true syndrome or disorder, this estimate could be lower than 1 percent of all MTBI patients.

Shedding new light on the true epidemiology of PCS raises an interesting comparison. Clinical lore has long held the assumption that brain neuroimaging is completely normal with no signs of structural injury in an overwhelming majority of MTBI cases. This assumption is sometimes taken to the extent of clinicians holding the position that a CT scan has little or no value in the case of concussion without any other signs of neurosurgical emergency because of the extremely low probability of yielding any clinically significant findings that would assist in diagnosis and alter treatment. As noted above, however, prospective controlled studies now demonstrate that as many as 10 percent of all patients with a Glasgow Coma Scale of 13–15 and meeting other diagnostic criteria for MTBI indeed have signs of structural injury detectable on head CT, brain MRI, or other advanced neuroimaging techniques. In contrast, clinical lore has also held that as many as 15–20 percent of all MTBI patients will follow a course of protracted recovery with persistent subjective complaints and poor functional outcome that will eventually warrant the diagnosis of persistent PCS.

Although estimates of abnormal imaging after MTBI and the true epidemiology of PCS are affected by the same issues of varied diagnostic criteria, research methodologies, and other factors that affect the true denominator, the empirical literature now suggests that our perspective on these two issues has perhaps been backward. That is, research over the past decade suggests that the likelihood of structural injury identifiable on brain neuroimaging is actually considerably *higher* than the true incidence of persistent PCS. In fact, the rate of abnormal imaging during the acute injury phase is likely two to three times greater than the probability that an MTBI patient will eventuate to persistent PCS. If we consider the empirical literature suggesting that "complicated MTBI" with abnormal imaging increases the likelihood that a patient will not follow the typical course of recovery in a matter of days to weeks, it is actually quite impressive that the true incidence of PCS is far lower 10 percent.

This point also raises an important implication that supports the distinction between "complicated" and "uncomplicated" MTBI. That is, there is little or no empirical evidence to support a neurophysiologic or "organic" basis for persistent PCS in uncomplicated MTBI without any identifiable structural injury, but those with complicated MTBI may be at increased risk for persistent symptoms and cognitive dysfunction beyond three months postinjury. That said, still an overwhelming majority of patients even with complicated MTBI follow a course of complete symptom, cognitive, and functional recovery over a period of weeks to months, and an extremely low percentage are diagnosed with persistent PCS.

Conclusion

Based on the scientific evidence, we now move closer to answering the original question as to whether or not persistent symptoms and other subjective complaints following MTBI are attributable to neurologic, psychological, or other, non-injury-related factors. Our ability to provide an evidence-based response to that question is imperative to developing effective PCS treatment interventions that ultimately improve functional outcome and reduce disability associated with MTBI.

18

■■■

PCS as a Neuropsychological Disorder

While the pathophysiology of MTBI itself is now well delineated and provides a clear neurologic basis for the acute symptoms and functional effects during the first several days to weeks postinjury, the base of scientific evidence makes it very unlikely that PCS is a neurologic condition stemming from an MTBI. That said, differential diagnosis of PCS still presents significant challenge to the clinician.

If Not PCS, What Else Could It Be?

As noted in preceding chapters, PCS-like symptoms can arise in a whole host of medical or psychological conditions, and the subjective complaints that define PCS can in some instances be influenced purposefully by motivational and other factors, particularly when there is potential for financial or other secondary gain.

Several studies have documented the connection between depression, anxiety, and stress during the acute phase after head injury in predicting the severity of postconcussion symptoms three months and further out from injury.[25] *Preexisting* psychiatric disturbance and psychological problems have also been found to complicate recovery after MTBI and increase the likelihood of persistent PCS.[26–30]

Several other demographic and psychosocial factors are also known to be associated with chronic PCS symptomatology, including female gender, older age, social difficulties, and environmental stress.[27,31–33] There is a significant association between somatic conditions of chronic pain, sleep disturbance, and persistent postconcussive symptoms.[1,34,35]

Iverson et al.[1] provide an exhaustive review on the importance of differential diagnosis and identifying various comorbidities that may erroneously lead to a patient being diagnosed with PCS. They concluded that the basis for persistent PCS is almost always "biopsychosocial," combining the acute neurologic effects of MTBI and a host of influential psychosocial factors, all of which are best suited for psychological and/or psychiatric treatment.[1]

Vanderploeg et al.[34] draw the following conclusion regarding the influence of psychological factors in PCS:

> The evidence reviewed reveals that although the injury to the brain sustained in an MTBI, as indicated by altered consciousness, plays a role in the experience of PCS, the development of PCS, is in large part, dependent on self expectations regarding the likely effects of an MTBI. In addition, the presence of PCS is mediated by factors such as individual resilience (cognitive reserve), preexisting psychological status, and psychosocial support.

Larrabee[36] offered that a persistence of "postconcussive" complaints is considered a function of *somatization*, which is potentially amenable to effective cognitive behavioral treatments. In a clinical setting, the concept of somatization is captured mainly in somatoform disorders, a group of disorders in which the common feature is the presence of physical (or, in the case of MTBI and PCS, also cognitive) symptoms that suggest a general medical condition (hence, the term somatoform) and are not fully explained by a general medical condition, but rather by the direct effects of a substance, or by another mental disorder (e.g., depression, anxiety, psychosis).[3] The symptoms of somatoform disorders are not intentionally produced and therefore are distinct from malingering and other factitious disorders that involve a purposeful and conscious feigning of symptoms or disabilities. If we consider PCS within the framework of a neuropsychological disorder, then diagnostically, the basis, symptoms, and course of PCS are likely most consistent with the DSM-IV criteria for undifferentiated somatoform disorder, which is characterized by unexplained symptoms (physical, cognitive) lasting at least six months, but typically below the threshold for diagnosis of somatization disorder.[3] Others have pointed out the overlap between PCS and posttraumatic stress disorder, linked not only by a common precipitating event in many cases, but also by a similar profile of subjective complaints.[1,37]

Other studies have investigated the influence of secondary gain or financial incentive on the maintenance of PCS symptoms. In their meta-analytic review,

Binder and Rohling[38] found the effect of financial incentive on outcome following MTBI to be quite significant (effect size = 0.47). Iverson et al.[1] also provide a detailed summary of the effects of litigation stress, exaggeration, and malingering on the maintenance of PCS. They conclude that

> exaggeration is very common in people believed to have a persistent post-concussive disorder who are being evaluated in relation to Workers Compensation claim, disability evaluation, or personal injury litigation. Malingering is much less common than exaggeration, and it would be a mistake to assume, without careful deliberation, that the exaggeration reflects malingering.

Conclusion

We have now reached a point where an abundance of scientific evidence and a clinical experience of experts in the field converge on an evidence-based conclusion that PCS should be considered and classified as a *neuropsychological* disorder. That is, while the neuropathophysiologic effects of MTBI start this process in motion, the development and maintenance of persistent PCS are more directly the result of psychological, psychosocial, and other non-MTBI-specific factors. Diagnostically, PCS is most reflective of published criteria for somatoform disorders, but may be confounded by separate or coexisting posttraumatic stress disorder. This empirically based (as opposed to nonspecific-symptom-based) perspective on PCS as a neuropsychological disorder requires the delineation of specific psychological principles underlying the disorder, which are summarized in chapter 19.

19

■ ■ ■

Psychological Theories of Postconcussion Syndrome

Over the past decade, several models describing the influence of psychological, social, personality, and motivational factors on persistent PCS have been either developed or refined. The most developed theories include the expectation as etiology theory,[39] the "good old days" theory,[40] the nocebo effect,[41] and a diasthesis-stress paradigm.[42] The common thread of these theories is their attempt to uncover the principles that predict the great variability in how people psychologically respond to MTBI and are predisposed to PCS.

Expectation as Etiology

The expectation as etiology theory[39] suggests that the incidence and persistence of PCS may be explained by the degree to which an individual misattributes common complaints to a prior head injury. For example, a patient may begin attributing all headaches to the head injury, despite a preinjury prevalence of headaches. In this regard, everyday complaints become linked to the injury, fuel the patient's expectations about the potential for long-term problems associated with head injury, and thus become more difficult to treat.

In their original study of this theory, Mittenberg et al.[39] administered a checklist of affective, somatic, and memory symptoms to 223 community volunteers who had no personal experience or knowledge of head injury and a clinically referred group of 100 head injury patients. Subjects indicated their current experiences of symptoms and then imagined having sustained a mild head injury in a motor vehicle accident and endorsed symptoms they expected to experience six months after their injury. The injured sample purported actual symptoms following their head injury. Imaginary concussion reliably showed expectations in controls of a coherent cluster of symptoms virtually identical to the postconcussion symptoms reported by patients with head trauma. Patients consistently underestimated the premorbid prevalence of these symptoms compared with the base rate in controls.

Mittenberg and colleagues concluded that symptom expectations appear to share as much variance with PCS as the head injury itself, thus leading to the "expectation as etiology" theory of PCS. The authors refute the assumption that cerebral dysfunction is the principal etiology for PCS symptoms and assert that their findings suggest that the principal etiology is the anticipation, widely held by individuals who have had no opportunity to observe or experience postconcussive symptoms, that PCS will occur following MTBI.

"Good Old Days" Hypothesis

Gunstad and Suhr[40] point out that the expectation as etiology theory fails to address the possibility that all individuals, not only those with documented head injuries, report experiencing more current symptoms than they experienced in the past. They point out the work of Ross and Conway,[43] who developed a constructive model of memory suggesting that individuals anchor memories on their current belief, attitude, or mood state and then infer information about the past in a manner consistent with their expectations.

Alternatively, Gunstad and Surh offer the "good old days" hypothesis, based on evidence that the "expectation as etiology" hypotheses may be too specific and that, following any negative event, people may attribute all symptoms to that negative event, regardless of a preexisting history of that very problem or other factors that may be influencing that problem.

In a 2001 study, Gunstad and Suhr[40] administered a PCS symptom checklist to 141 research participants that included normal controls, healthy athletes, and depressed individuals. Participants were asked to rate their current symptoms and symptoms expected following a hypothetical MTBI. Head-injured athletes, chronic headache sufferers, and a second sample of normal controls reported current symptoms and retrospective symptoms (prior to their injury/illness or for some point in the past). Depressed individuals reported more current symptoms than did normal controls and healthy athletes, demonstrating that PCS symptoms are not specific to PCS. All groups expected more symptoms following mild head injury than currently experienced, supporting the idea that individuals expect negative consequence following head injury. However, healthy athletes expected fewer symptoms than did normals or depressed individuals, possibly due to pre-existing expectations for speedy recovery. Both head-injured athletes and headache sufferers reported more current symptoms than the past, but not at a rate lower than the baseline for normal controls.

This tendency of people to recall past symptoms and functioning more favorably than was actually the case is further complicated by involvement and personal head injury litigation.[1] A response bias is sometimes observed in symptom recall by plaintiffs compared to nonlitigants. Studies have demonstrated that personal injury claimants free from head trauma tend to report a lower preaccident prevalence of cognitive, mental, and emotional symptoms in their daily lives compared to nonlitigants.[44,45]

Nocebo Effect

Another model suggesting a possible cognitive mechanism for PCS is the nocebo effect,[41] which is a more specific rendering of Kirsch's response expectation theory.[46] Response expectations are "anticipations of automatic reactions to particular situational cues" and are outside both volition and conscious thought.[40] In basic terms, the nocebo effect applies when expectations of sickness and associated emotional distress cause the sickness in question. Iverson et al.[1] concluded that the nocebo effect in general, and expectations regarding symptoms and problems associated with MTBI in particular, likely represents significant psychological factors in the perception and reporting of PCS symptoms.

Gunstad and Suhr[14] conducted a study on the perception of illness and nonspecificity of PCS symptoms expectations. Their study suggested that individuals do not expect a specific constellation of symptoms following head injury, because individuals portraying head injury, posttraumatic stress, and depression expected similar number and types of symptoms. They concluded that their findings were consistent with the predictions of the "good old days" model and a generalized nocebo effect, because both models predict individuals would expect nonspecific negative consequences from an undesirable event.

Diasthesis-Stress Model

Wood[42] offers a diasthesis-stress paradigm that examines the interaction between physiologic and psychological factors that generate and maintain postconcussional symptoms. Wood's theory includes that motivational factors and different coping strategies explain why some people are at risk of developing PCS. Iatrogenic forces can also influence a patient's recovery after MTBI, particularly if health care providers inadvertently reinforce misperceptions of symptoms or insecurities about recovery. An unfortunate scenario unfolds when a patient with vague symptom complaints and no clear indication of significant head trauma is told he has "brain damage" and will never make a complete neurologic, symptom, or functional recovery. The long-term damage of creating that perception for a patient is most difficult to undo. Wood added that the rationale and effectiveness of interventions that ameliorate the impact of early postconcussional symptoms are most critical to prevention of PCS.

Conclusion

In summary, individual cases of persistent PCS are likely fueled by a combination of core principles from the various psychological theories of PCS.[47] Clarifying the specific psychological mechanisms underlying PCS in turn provide the basis of effective methods for intervention and treatment, as discussed in chapter 20.

20

■■■

Interventional Models for Postconcussion Syndrome

The main implication from the evidence that PCS represents a psychological disorder is its reversibility in most cases with effective psychological treatment. From the psychological theories of PCS have also come well-developed interventional models to remediate PCS symptoms and return the patient to preinjury functional levels.

Several studies have investigated the influence of early psychological intervention and treatment for MTBI, most of which rely on principles of cognitive-behavioral therapy and effective patient education. At least one group of experts has actually developed a therapist manual for cognitive-behavioral treatment of PCS.[48]

Efficacy of Interventional Models

In a 1996 study, Mittenberg et al.[49] investigated the cognitive behavioral prevention of PCS. A treatment group of 29 MTBI patients received a printed manual and met with a therapist prior to hospital discharge to review the nature and incidence of expected symptoms, the cognitive-behavioral model of symptom maintenance and treatment, techniques for reducing symptoms, and instructions for gradual resumption of premorbid activities. A control group of 29 MTBI patients received routine hospital treatment and discharge instructions. All patients in both groups had MTBI with a Glasgow Coma Scale score of 13–15 on admission without any measurable period of post-traumatic amnesia. Subjects were randomly assigned to the treatment or control group, and there were no differences between the groups on demographic or injury-related characteristics. At six months postinjury, patients were contacted by an interviewer who was blinded to their group assignment.

The results from this study demonstrated that treated patients reported significantly shorter average symptom duration (33 vs. 51 days) and significantly fewer of the 12 symptoms at follow-up (1.6 vs. 3.1). Subjects were also asked how much each symptom had occurred in the previous week and to rate the severity of each symptom. The treatment group experienced significantly fewer symptomatic days (0.5 vs. 1.3) and lower mean severity levels. The investigators concluded that their results suggest that brief, early psychological intervention can indeed reduce the incidence of PCS. These results also indicate that the treated group had a symptom level essentially no higher than the base rate in a normal population, and the untreated group had a symptom level, on average, that technically approximates the required level in the DSM-IV and ICD-10 diagnostic criteria.

Ponsford et al.[50] evaluated the impact of providing information on outcome measured in terms of reported symptoms, cognitive performance, and psychological adjustment in children three months after injury. Sixty-one children with MTBI were assessed one week and three months after injury, and 58 children with MTBI were assessed three months after injury only. They were compared with two control groups ($n = 45$ and 47) of children with minor injuries not involving the head. Participants completed measures of preinjury behavior and psychological adjustment, postconcussion symptoms, and tests of attention, speed of information processing, and memory. Children with MTBI seen at one week were also given an information booklet outlining symptoms associated with MTBI and suggested coping strategies, which served as the intervention in this particular study. Those seen only at three months after injury did not receive this booklet.

Their results indicated that children with MTBI reported more symptoms than controls at one week but demonstrated no impairments on neuropsychological measures. Initial symptoms had resolved for most children by three months after injury, but a small group of children who had previous head injury or a history of learning or behavioral difficulties reported ongoing problems. The group not seen at one week and not given the information booklet reported more symptoms overall and were more stressed three months after injury. Ponsford et al.[50] concluded that providing an informational booklet reduces anxiety and thereby lowers the incidence of ongoing problems associated with MTBI and PCS.

In 2004, Kashluba et al.[51] conducted a longitudinal, controlled study of patient complaints following treated MTBI. The study provided three-month follow-up data to a previous study that compared symptom complaints of patients with MTBI with those of noninjured control participants within one month of injury. One hundred ten MTBI patients and 118 control participants were grouped matched on age, gender, educational level, and socioeconomic status. As a group, MTBI patients no longer endorsed significantly more symptoms than did the control group. Only 3 of the 43 queried symptoms were endorsed by significantly more MTBI patients than controls. Overall, the treated MTBI group symptom complaints diminished from baseline to three months postinjury, with relatively few differences remaining between the two groups.

The WHO Collaborating Centre Task Force on Mild Traumatic Brain Injury examined the totality of evidence for nonsurgical interventions and for economic cost for MTBI patients by a systematic search of the literature and a best-evidence synthesis.[6,52] After screening 38,806 abstracts, WHO critically reviewed 45 articles on intervention and accepted 16 (36 percent). They eventually reviewed 16 articles on economic costs and accepted seven of them (44 percent). In conclusion, the task force findings supported the findings of the aforementioned individual studies by declaring that early educational information can reduce long-term complaints and that this early intervention need not be intensive.

Conclusion

To summarize, several studies have demonstrated that supportive psychological and educational interventions can effectively reduce the incidence of PCS, which in turn enhances functional outcome and alleviates the burden of disability associated with MTBI. These interventions need not be intensive and are most effective when introduced early during the acute or subacute recovery phase after MTBI.

21

███

A Practical Model for Clinical Management of PCS

In this progression toward transferring scientific evidence to clinical application, I now present a strong foundation of theory and research on interventional models for treating PCS as a neuropsychological disorder. To reiterate, the construct of "neuropsychological disorder" is based on the fact that MTBI and PCS, perhaps more than any other entity in neuroscience, call on a clinician's expert understanding of both neurologic and psychological principals. While there is little question about the neuropathophysiology of MTBI, it is the clinician's understanding of psychological principals that will be most effective in treating the individual patient who presents with lingering complaints or other difficulties after MTBI that eventuate to a diagnosis of persistent PCS.

Role of the Neuropsychologist

Here is where I must *again* acknowledge my bias not only that is PCS uniquely a neuropsychological disorder, but also that neuropsychologists are the clinicians best suited to evaluate and treat MTBI and PCS. This assertion assumes that the vital assignments of the neurologist and neurosurgeon have already been completed in ruling out any underlying neurosurgical emergency or other conditions that would warrant emergent medical treatment. I also suspect that neurologists, neurosurgeons, and other physicians would be delighted by the offer of neuropsychologists to take the lead in managing the rather complicated care of their MTBI patients.

Historically, the role of the neuropsychologist following MTBI has been restricted to evaluation of cognitive and other complaints and assisting in the differential diagnosis of PCS. There is no question as to the value of a thorough evaluation by an expertly trained neuropsychologist given the complexity in the differential diagnosis of PCS. Objective measurement of subjective cognitive complaints is most crucial to documenting and tracking cognitive recovery after MTBI, as well as guiding treatment planning as to the need for any occupational, academic, or other restrictions/accommodations based on the patients cognitive functioning during the acute phase after their injury.

Beyond the acute MTBI phase, the trained neuropsychologist should be aware of all factors and comorbidities that may contribute to the presentation of PCS-like symptoms and consider any and all in the differential diagnosis. Most crucial is an awareness of the nonspecificity of PCS-like symptoms that may manifest in a whole assortment of medical and psychological conditions separate from MTBI and PCS.

In most settings, the challenge for clinicians and patients comes at the point of providing systematic, effective treatment for MTBI and PCS patients. This includes the evaluating neuropsychologist whose practice often does not extend beyond neuropsychological assessment to intervention and treatment, whether it be for PCS or other neurologic or psychological conditions.

Hospital-Based Model for Clinical Management of MTBI

I close this text with presentation of a practical, evidence-based interventional model for MTBI and PCS. In keeping with the recommendations of the WHO Collaborating Centre Task Force on Mild Traumatic Brain Injury,[52] this model is based on the principle that effective intervention must be early, easily accessible, supportive, educational, and anchored in the empirical literature. Also in keeping with the WHO recommendations, this interventional model is not intensive in terms of sophisticated neurologic workup, advanced neuroimaging, or aggressive medical treatment.

Several institutions around the United States have implemented MTBI assessment protocols and PCS treatment models, most of which are led by a clinical neuropsychologist and a partnering physician expert either emergency medicine, neurology, neurosurgery, or physiatry.

The MTBI intervention model presented here capitalizes on the first point of patient contact by emergency medical service (EMS) professionals and hospital emergency department personnel. Like many similar models around the country, the MTBI team is mainly composed of a physiatrist, neuropsychologist, and nurse coordinator. This core group has teamed with emergency medicine physicians to educate local EMS on the assessment and management of TBI. Our group has provided some EMS crews with screening tools for rapid assessment of symptoms and cognitive functioning in the MTBI patient. In some instances, EMS groups have also collaborated on TBI research initiatives directed by our group. This has created an invaluable link with our local first responders who triage TBI, including MTBI, in the field.

Perhaps the most vital link in the chain of care for MTBI patients comes at the hospital emergency department. Similar to our efforts with EMS crews, our core MTBI group also offers education and ongoing consultation to the emergency department physicians and staff. This activity has ranged from in-service training to providing educational materials for staff and patients. Figure 21.1 shows a TBI Fact Card and Box 21.1 displays an informational sheet on MTBI, both of which our group developed for emergency department staff to distribute to TBI patients upon discharge. We also make these materials available to primary care physicians and specialists that see MTBI patients who did not receive care at the hospital emergency department. You will note that both forms include information on how to contact our TBI clinic for any patient in need of follow-up care or other supportive resources after their injury.

The key to efficient operation of our clinic is the TBI program coordinator, a registered nurse with background in neurosurgical and neurologic critical care. The coordinator is an invaluable liaison to the emergency department and referring physicians, while also providing a direct point of care coordination for TBI patients. The coordinator triages referrals to the TBI clinic and assesses the potential role of the physiatrist, neuropsychologist, or other specialists in the patient's care.

Multidisciplinary Approach

Our TBI clinic takes a multidisciplinary approach to evaluation and treatment of MTBI. The clinic is designed to accommodate TBI referrals during the acute phase (1–5 days) of injury, in keeping with the WHO recommendation that intervention for MTBI is most effective when delivered early. The role of the TBI program coordinator is also vital in this regard, as she provides a direct point of contact for referrals (sometimes by a call directly from the emergency department before the patient is released) and can quickly coordinate the initial clinic visit when the neuropsychologist and physiatrist will jointly evaluate the patient and provide treatment recommendations.

Before the first clinic visit, the coordinator collects extensive information on the patient's injury and general history, while also securing relevant records and diagnostic studies. The initial clinic visit typically involves a brief evaluation by the neuropsychologist, including an MTBI symptom checklist

OUTPATIENT
— CONCUSSION & BRAIN —
INJURY CLINIC

ProHealth Care's Neuroscience Center is pleased to introduce its new outpatient Concussion and Brain Injury Clinic. This specialty clinic is designed to provide follow-up evaluation and treatment during the acute phase after an emergency room visit or hospitalization due to concussion or more severe traumatic brain injury.

◆ **The Hard Facts on Head Injury**

Traumatic brain injury (TBI) is the largest cause of disability and death among young people in the United States every year. More than 75% of head injuries are mild and involve no loss of consciousness, *but can result in significant symptoms and lingering functional deficits that warrant further evaluation and treatment, including:*

- Headache
- Dizziness
- Nausea
- Vomiting
- Disorientation
- Light-headedness
- Sensitivity to light and noise

- Poor concentration
- Memory problems
- Fatigue
- Irritability
- Depression
- Anxiety
- Sleep problems

◆ **Early Intervention Makes the Difference**

The goal of our outpatient clinic is to provide individualized evaluation and treatment *during the acute phase* after head injury in a medical model proven to maximize recovery and reduce disability associated with head injury and Post–Concussive Syndrome.

For More Information

For More Information about the clinic or to refer a patient, call Deb Swearingen, RN. TBI Program Coordinator at (262) 928-8200.

continued on reverse

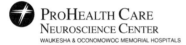

PROHEALTH CARE
NEUROSCIENCE CENTER
WAUKESHA & OCONOMOWOC MEMORIAL HOSPITALS

ProHealth Care's Concussion and Brain Injury Clinic will directly benefit patients and their treating physicians through:

◆ **Collaboration with Primary Care Physician:**
The patient's care will be closely coordinated with primary care and other treating physicians. A detailed report of diagnostic results and treatment recommendations will be provided to ensure continuity of care.

◆ **Expert Physicians and Staff Provide Individualized Treatment:**
Medical direction is provided by Julie Wilson, MD. physical medicine and rehabilitation specialist. The team of specialists from the WMH Neuropsychology Service will provide consultation to more formally evaluate deficits and recovery after TBI. Other members of the multidisciplinary team include:
- Rehabilitation Therapies (Physical, occupational and speech therapy)
- Behavioral Medicine to address depression, anxiety and psychological effects of TBI

◆ **Dedicated Care Coordinator:**
A program coordinator will provide support and education, help patients navigate through follow-up care and ensure continuity of care as the "go to person" for patients and others in need of TBI resources.

◆ **Evidence-Based Approach to Treatment:**
Waukesha Memorial Hospital has been home to a nationally-respected clinical research program studying the effects of concussion. Applied research aimed at identifying factors that enhance clinical outcomes after head injury will continue to be a key component of the Concussion and Brain Injury Clinic.

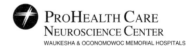

PROHEALTH CARE
NEUROSCIENCE CENTER
WAUKESHA & OCONOMOWOC MEMORIAL HOSPITALS

FIGURE 21.1. Sample "TBI Fact Card" for Health Care Providers and Patients.

and abbreviated cognitive battery focused on assessing memory, cognitive processing speed, and other functions most sensitive to deficit after MTBI. The neuropsychologist then consults with the coordinator and physiatrist on findings from the neuropsychological examination and treatment options before providing the patient (and family) immediate feedback and recommendations. The physiatrist typically evaluates the patient from the standpoint of any injuries requiring physical rehabilitation or medical treatment (e.g., antidepressant, mood stabilizer, sleep agent).

BOX 21.1 Informational Guide for MTBI Patients

Recovering from Mild Head Injury/Concussion: A Guide for Patients

Mild head injury/concussion is a relatively common injury, which typically occurs from a blow to the head during sports, an accident, or a fall. People often report being dazed or knocked unconscious for a short period of time from their injury. People also frequently report brief memory loss for events just before, during, or immediately following the injury. This is common and not a cause for concern. Although many people do not seek treatment after injury, it is common for people to present to the emergency room for evaluation. A typical evaluation in the ER may include a brain scan and thorough medical examination to rule out a more serious head injury.

Common Symptoms

You should not be alarmed if you have some symptoms after mild head injury. Some symptoms are expected. As noted, feeling dazed, being knocked unconscious, or having amnesia for events that happened before or after the injury are very common indicators of mild head injury. Most patients will also have some temporary symptoms associated with their head injury that may persist for a short time after the injury. Common temporary symptoms may include headache, blurry or double vision, sensitivity to bright light, fatigue, reduced concentration or memory complaints, irritability, or other mood changes like depression or anxiety. Few patients will experience all postconcussive symptoms.

Duration of Symptoms

Most symptoms following a mild head injury/concussion resolve in a short period of time, from days, weeks, or up to a few months, even without treatment. Symptoms persisting longer than 3 to 6 months are quite rare following mild head injury. It is also important to keep in mind that postconcussive symptoms (e.g., headache, memory lapses) are experienced by all individuals from time to time in their

(continued)

daily lives, so one should not expect that recovery means a person will never experience these symptoms after head injury. Recovery is better defined as returning to your preinjury baseline.

Treatment

The goal of treatment is to help you understand the injury more thoroughly, develop appropriate appraisal of symptoms postinjury, and develop appropriate expectations about symptom resolution and recovery. Having accurate self-appraisals and appropriate expectations about recovery will help you manage symptoms much more effectively as you recover. Symptom management may include temporary lifestyle or behavioral changes or medications recommended or prescribed by your doctor. Treatment will ideally help you return to activities (e.g., work, exercise, school, etc.) in a timely manner.

Your doctors and health care providers will work with you to help you manage your symptoms as you recover from your injury. They will tailor their recommendations based on your background (i.e., medical history) and current symptoms to help maximize your quality of life during your recovery and your return to activities such as work or school in a timely fashion.

Follow-up

Although follow-up in our clinic or referral to other specialists may be recommended to help monitor or manage symptoms, it is not always necessary. If it is felt that you do not need follow-up or referral for symptom management after your visit, we still encourage you to contact us in the future with any new questions or concerns. If your questions cannot be addressed with a phone call, we could see you back in our clinic if necessary or refer you to a provider that could best address your needs.

Please call our TBI Coordinator at 262-928-8200 if you have any questions or concerns about your recovery.

Educational material adapted from Mittenberg W, Fischera S. Recovery from Mild Head Injury: A treatment manual for patients. *Psychotherapy in Private Practice* 1993;12:37-52, with permission.

A follow-up care plan is arranged based on the patient's care needs, typically involving brief follow-up with the neuropsychologist, physiatrist, or both. The main intervention delivered by the core group is educational and psychological in most cases. Medical treatment is prescribed in a smaller percentage of cases. Our TBI program coordinator also provides interim supportive follow-up to patients over the course of their recovery. In most instances, patients are seen for one or two visits after their initial evaluation, when their progress is evaluated. Follow-up visits consist mostly of reassurance, continued education, and addressing factors (e.g., psychological, social, medical) potentially interfering with recovery.

We do not yet have empirical data to test the efficacy of our model on outcome, but we plan to do so, much like other interventional programs have measured elsewhere. Anecdotally, we have been pleased with the response of both referring physicians and patients to our TBI clinic initiative. Again, emergency medicine physicians and other health care providers appreciate a systematic model of follow-up so that MTBI patients do not "fall through the cracks." This point was embraced more wholeheartedly when we presented to our referring community the compelling evidence on how early intervention and education ultimately improve outcomes for individual patients after MTBI. Patients also clearly appreciate the services provided by our coordinator, neuropsychologist, and physiatrist who provide a thorough assessment of the injury and coordinated care to maximize their recovery. Finally, as neuropsychologists, it has been quite refreshing to consult on MTBI cases very early during the acute and subacute recovery phase when intervention has the greatest chance of improving outcome, rather than the classic scenario of evaluating the "refractory" PCS patient months after injury.

Conclusion

In summary, putting the correct resources in place can result in a practical approach to clinical management of MTBI and PCS in most hospital settings. The triad of nursing coordinator, neuropsychologist, and physician with specialized interest in TBI provides a valuable resource to both health care professionals and TBI patients. Developing connections with EMS and the hospital emergency department is key in order to expedite acute MTBI referrals who will benefit most from early intervention. The neuropsychologist's role is somewhat nontraditional in applying brief cognitive assessment methods appropriate for evaluating MTBI during the acute phase, as opposed to the lengthier traditional battery. The multidisciplinary model of neuropsychologist and physician jointly caring for the MTBI patient not only provides clinical value but also is more efficient and convenient for the patient. In the end, this interventional model shows great promise in reducing the incidence of PCS and improving overall outcome for our local MTBI patients.

Part Four Top 10 Conclusions

1. Symptom-based diagnosis of PCS is plagued by several factors, most notably poor reliability of diagnostic criteria and nonspecificity of PCS symptoms.

2. Symptoms that make up the core criteria for the formal diagnosis of PCS are also highly nonspecific to either MTBI or PCS and are commonly reported in psychiatric disorders, medical illness, and even healthy individuals.

3. Estimates suggesting that 15–20 percent of MTBI patients have persistent PCS or disorder are severely inflated; the true incidence of PCS is more likely in the range of 1–5 percent of all MTBI patients.

4. Contrary to conventional thought, the frequency of structural injury identifiable on brain neuroimaging after acute MTBI may actually be considerably *higher* than the true incidence of persistent PCS.

5. The base of scientific evidence directs us toward rethinking PCS as a neuropsychological disorder associated with the transient neurologic effects of MTBI but maintained by a combination of psychological and social factors in the overwhelming majority of cases.

6. A combination of psychological principles related to expectations of recovery and iatrogenic factors contribute to individual cases of persistent PCS.

7. Exaggeration of symptoms or subjective functional complaints should be ruled out in cases of persistent PCS with potential for secondary gain; symptom exaggeration is typically

multifactorial in nature, but does not automatically reflect malingering, which is much less common.

8. Supportive psychological and educational interventions can effectively reduce the incidence of PCS.

9. Existing treatment models for PCS are proven to enhances functional outcome and reduce disability associated with MTBI.

10. Putting the correct resources in place can result in a practical approach to clinical management of MTBI and PCS that provides great value to health care providers and patients in most hospital settings.

References

1. Iverson GL, Zasler ND, Lange RT. Post-concussive disorder. In: Zasler ND, Katz DI, Zafonte RD, eds. *Brain Injury Medicine: Principles and Practice*. New York: Demos Medical Publishing, 2006; 373–405.

2. World Health Organization. *International Statistical Classification of Diseases and Related Health Problems*, 10th ed. Geneva, Switzerland: World Health Organization, 1992.

3. American Psychological Association. *Diagnostic and Statistical Manual of Mental Disorders*, 4th ed. Washington, DC: American Psychiatric Association, 1994.

4. Boake C, McCauley SR, Levin HS, et al. Limited agreement between criteria-based diagnoses of postconcussional syndrome. *J Neuropsychiatry Clin Neurosci* 2004;16:493–99.

5. Boake C, McCauley SR, Levin HS, et al. Diagnostic criteria for postconcussional syndrome after mild to moderate traumatic brain injury. *J Neuropsychiatry Clin Neurosci* 2005;17:350–56.

6. Carroll LJ, Cassidy JD, Peloso PM, et al. Prognosis for mild traumatic brain injury: results of the WHO Collaborating Centre Task Force on Mild Traumatic Brain Injury. *J Rehabil Med* 2004; 43:84–105.

7. McCauley SR, Boake C, Pedroza C, et al. Postconcussional disorder: are the DSM-IV criteria an improvement over the ICD-10? *J Nerv Ment Dis* 2005;193:540–50.

8. Kashluba S, Casey JE, Paniak C. Evaluating the utility of ICD-10 diagnostic criteria for postconcussion syndrome following mild traumatic brain injury. *J Int Neuropsychol Soc* 2006;12:111–18.

9. Sawchyn JM, Brulot MM, Strauss E. Note on the use of the postconcussion syndrome checklist. *Arch Clin Neuropsychol* 2000;15:1–8.

10. Radanov BP, Dvorak J, Valach L. Cognitive deficits in patients after soft tissue injury of the cervical spine. *Spine* 1992;17:127–31.

11. Trahan DE, Ross CE, Trahan SL. Relationships among postconcussional-type symptoms, depression, and anxiety in neurologically normal young adults and victims of mild brain injury. *Arch Clin Neuropsychol* 2001;16:435–45.

12. Dunn JT, Lees-Haley PR, Brown RS, Williams CW, English LT. Neurotoxic complaint base rates of personal injury claimants: implications for neuropsychological assessment. *J Clin Psychol* 1995; 51:577–84.

13. Ingebrigtsen T, Waterloo K, Marup-Jensen S, Attner E, Romner B. Quantification of post-concussion symptoms 3 months after minor head injury in 100 consecutive patients. *J Neurol* 1998;245:609–12.

14. Gunstad J, Suhr JA. Perception of illness: nonspecificity of postconcussion syndrome symptom expectation. *J Int Neuropsychol Soc* 2002;8:37–47.

15. Wang Y, Chan RC, Deng Y. Examination of postconcussion-like symptoms in healthy university students: relationships to subjective and objective neuropsychological function performance. *Arch Clin Neuropsychol* 2006;21:339–47.

16. Iverson GL, Lange RT. Examination of "postconcussion-like" symptoms in a healthy sample. *Appl Neuropsychol* 2003;10:137–44.

17. Iverson GL. Misdiagnosis of the persistent postconcussion syndrome in patients with depression. *Arch Clin Neuropsychol* 2006;21:303–10.

18. Lees-Haley PR, Fox DD, Courtney JC. A comparison of complaints by mild brain injury claimants and other claimants describing subjective experiences immediately following their injury. *Arch Clin Neuropsychol* 2001;16:689–95.

19. Suhr JA, Gunstad J. Postconcussive symptom report: the relative influence of head injury and depression. *J Clin Exp Neuropsychol* 2002;24:981–93.

20. Alexander MP. Mild traumatic brain injury: pathophysiology, natural history, and clinical management. *Neurology* 1995;45:1253–60.

21. Rutherford WH, Merrett JD, McDonald JR. Symptoms at one year following concussion from minor head injuries. *Injury* 1979;10:225–30.

22. McLean A Jr, Temkin NR, Dikmen S, Wyler AR. The behavioral sequelae of head injury. *J Clin Neuropsychol* 1983;5:361–76.

23. Alves W, Macciocchi SN, Barth JT. Post-concussive symptoms after uncomplicated head injury. *J Head Trauma Rehabil* 1993;8:48–59.

24. Iverson GL. Outcome from mild traumatic brain injury. *Curr Opin Psychiatry* 2005;18:301–17.

25. King NS. Emotional, neuropsychological, and organic factors: their use in the prediction of persisting postconcussion symptoms after moderate and mild head injuries. *J Neurol Neurosurg Psychiatry* 1996;61:75–81.

26. Binder LM, Rohling ML, Larrabee GJ. A review of mild head trauma. Part I: meta-analytic review of neuropsychological studies. *J Clin Exp Neuropsychol* 1997;19:421–31.

27. Fenton G, McClelland R, Montgomery A, MacFlynn G, Rutherford W. The postconcussional syndrome: social antecedents and psychological sequelae. *Br J Psychiatry* 1993;162:493–97.

28. Greiffenstein MF, Baker JW. Comparison of premorbid and post-injury MMPI-2 profiles in late postconcussion claimants. *Clin Neuropsychol* 2001;15:162–70.

29. Robertson E, Rath B, Fournet G, Zelhart P, Estes R. Assessment of mild brain trauma: a preliminary study of the influence of premorbid factors. *Clin Neuropsychol* 1994;8:69–74.

30. Fann JR, Katon WJ, Uomoto JM, Esselman PC. Psychiatric disorders and functional disability in outpatients with traumatic brain injuries. *Am J Psychiatry* 1995;152:1493–99.

31. Gouvier WD, Cubic B, Jones G, Brantley P, Cutlip Q. Postconcussion symptoms and daily stress in normal and head-injured college populations. *Arch Clin Neuropsychol* 1992;7:193–211.

32. Radanov BP, di Stefano G, Schnidrig A, Ballinari P. Role of psychosocial stress in recovery from common whiplash. *Lancet* 1991;338:712–15.

33. Santa Maria MP, Pinkston JB, Miller SR, Gouvier WD. Stability of postconcussion symptomatology differs between high and low responders and by gender but not by mild head injury status. *Arch Clin Neuropsychol* 2001;16:133–40.

34. Vanderploeg RD, Belanger HG, Curtiss G. Mild traumatic brain injury: medical and neuropsychological causality modeling. In: Young G, Kane A, Nicholson K, eds. *Psychological Knowledge in Court: PTSD, Pain and TBI*. New York: Springer-Verlag, 2006; 279–307.

35. Nicholson K. Pain, cognition and traumatic brain injury. *NeuroRehabilitation* 2000;14:95–103.

36. Larrabee GJ. Neuropsychological outcome, post concussion symptoms, and forensic considerations in mild closed head trauma. *Semin Clin Neuropsychiatry* 1997;2:196–206.

37. Harvey AG, Brewin CR, Jones C, Kopelman MD. Coexistence of posttraumatic stress disorder and traumatic brain injury: towards a resolution of the paradox. *J Int Neuropsychol Soc* 2003;9:663–76.

38. Binder LM, Rohling ML. Money matters: a meta-analytic review of the effects of financial incentives on recovery after closed-head injury. *Am J Psychiatry* 1996;153:7–10.

39. Mittenberg W, DiGiulio DV, Perrin S, Bass AE. Symptoms following mild head injury: expectation as aetiology. *J Neurol Neurosurg Psychiatry* 1992;55:200–4.

40. Gunstad J, Suhr JA. "Expectation as etiology" versus "the good old days": postconcussion syndrome symptom reporting in athletes, headache sufferers, and depressed individuals. *J Int Neuropsychol Soc* 2001;7:323–33.

41. Hahn RA. The nocebo phenomenon: concept, evidence, and implications for public health. *Prev Med* 1997;26:607–11.

42. Wood RL. Understanding the 'miserable minority': a diathesis-stress paradigm for post-concussional syndrome. *Brain Inj* 2004;18:1135–53.

43. Ross M, Conway M. Remembering one's own past: the construction of personal histories. In: Sorrentino RM, Higgens ET, eds. *Handbook of Motivation and Cognition. Vol. 1*. New York: Guilford Press, 1986; 122–44.

44. Lees-Haley PR, Williams CW, English LT. Response bias in self-reported history of plaintiffs compared with non-litigating patients. *Psychol Rep* 1996;79:811–18.

45. Lees-Haley PR, Williams CW, Zasler ND, Marguilies S, English LT, Stevens KB. Response bias in plaintiffs' histories. *Brain Inj* 1997;11: 791–99.

46. Kirsch I. Response expectancy as a determinant of experience and behavior. *Am Psychol* 1985;54:504–15.

47. Greiffenstein MF. Late post-concussion syndrome as a learned illness behavior: proposal for a multifactorial model. *Brain Inj Source* 2000;4:26–27.

48. Ferguson RJ, Mittenberg W. Cognitive-behavioral treatment of postconcussion syndrome. In: Van Hasselt VB, Hersen M, eds. *Sourcebook of Psychological Treatment Manuals for Adult Disorders.* New York: Plenum Press, 1996; 615–55.

49. Mittenberg W, Tremont G, Zielinski RE, Fichera S, Rayls KR. Cognitive-behavioral prevention of postconcussion syndrome. *Arch Clin Neuropsychol* 1996;11:139–45.

50. Ponsford J, Willmott C, Rothwell A, et al. Impact of early intervention on outcome after mild traumatic brain injury in children. *Pediatrics* 2001;108:1297–303.

51. Kashluba S, Paniak C, Blake T, Reynolds S, Toller-Lobe G, Nagy J. A longitudinal, controlled study of patient complaints following treated mild traumatic brain injury. *Arch Clin Neuropsychol* 2004;19:805–16.

52. Borg J, Holm L, Peloso PM, et al. Non-surgical intervention and cost for mild traumatic brain injury: results of the WHO Collaborating Centre Task Force on Mild Traumatic Brain Injury. *J Rehabil Med* 2004:76–83.

Final Summary and Conclusions

The science of mild traumatic brain injury (MTBI) and postconcussion syndrome (PCS) has advanced more in the past 10 years than in the prior several decades combined. Parts one through four of this text have highlighted the major breakthroughs over the past 5–10 years that have significantly increased our scientific understanding of the true incidence and impact, basic and clinical science, natural history, and outcome associated with MTBI, and it is my hope that this, in turn, provides us with an evidence base for clinical diagnosis and treatment.

There is little question that TBI is a major public health problem worldwide, regardless of the metric applied (incidence, death and disability, societal impact). The reality is that most TBIs fall into the mild category, which the literature clearly and consistently indicates is a different animal altogether from moderate and severe TBI. Not only have the complexities of MTBI made it difficult to prospectively study these injuries, but also the lack of research has made it difficult for clinicians seeking evidence-based approaches to the clinical management of MTBI. Thankfully, the research reviewed throughout this text translates readily and effectively to clinical practice for the diagnosis and treatment of both MTBI and PCS.

If we synthesize the information presented in parts one through four, a nicely integrated model of MTBI emerges. We now recognize a minimum biomechanical threshold necessary and sufficient to trigger the "neurometabolic cascade" that manifests as a combination of symptoms, cognitive dysfunction, and other functional deficits that are the hallmarks of MTBI, even in the absence of observed unconsciousness, lengthy amnesia, or focal neurologic deficits. The literature also clearly demonstrates, however, that a single, uncomplicated concussion is a transient neurologic event characterized by gradual resolution of symptoms, cognitive dysfunction, and complete recovery at a *brain level* (e.g., neurophysiologically) within days to weeks of injury. Fortunately for those affected, most MTBI patients resume their normal independent functioning soon after injury without complication.

Although still considered in the category of MTBI, those with more severe grades of injury characterized by focal brain lesions may follow a slower or less complete recovery course. Exposure to repeated MTBI may also alter the expected recovery course and may even create risk of long-term psychiatric and neurologic problems over a lifespan. This issue is particularly of great concern among amateur and professional athletes who suffer multiple MTBIs over their many years of participation in contact or collision sports.

The true incidence of persistent PCS after MTBI is likely much lower than has been previously reported in the literature, perhaps as low as 1–5 percent of all MTBI cases. Furthermore, PCS is fueled more by psychological, social, and motivational factors than acute injury characteristics of MTBI. Theory, research, and clinical practice all converge on the concept of PCS as a neuropsychological disorder associated with the acute, transient neurologic effects of MTBI but maintained by a host of non-injury-related factors in the overwhelming majority of cases.

Fortunately, PCS is highly treatable with supportive patient education and cognitive-behavioral therapy. In a clinical setting, a multidisciplinary approach to management of MTBI and PCS is most effective, particular when delivered by a core team consisting of physician, neuropsychologist, and nursing care coordinator. Applied research and clinical experience suggest that this approach not only is most appropriate to treating PCS but also improves functional outcome for MTBI patients, both of which go a long way to reducing the overall public health burden associated with MTBI.

In closing, I hope this text presents researchers with an integrated index of the important work in MTBI over the past decade and offers health care providers the evidence base that I have been seeking to drive my strategies for clinical management of MTBI and PCS.

Index

Page numbers followed by "f" denote figures; those followed by "t" denote tables; and those followed by "b" denote boxes

Posttraumatic amnesia
  description of, 18, 46–47, 58
  duration of, 165
Posttraumatic amnesia (*continued*)
  recovery affected by, 119–123
  studies of, 119–123
Posttraumatic stress disorder, 170
Prognosis
  information gaps in, 30
  WHO Collaborating Centre Task
    Force findings, 85–86, 131
Project Sideline, 87–95

Race, 5
Recovery. *See also* Outcomes
  cognitive. *See* Cognitive recovery
  diffusion tensor imaging predictions,
    65
  iatrogenic factors, 176
  information gaps in, 30
  injury severity correlated with, 129
  loss of consciousness and, 121
  neurophysiologic, 125–128
  posttraumatic amnesia and, 121
  psychological factors that affect, 109,
    131, 169
  subacute phase, 127
  summary of, 132
Recurrent MTBI
  cumulative effects of, 134
  longitudinal studies of, 36–37
  memory performance after, 136
  outcomes affected by, 196
  of sport-related concussion, 35–36
  studies of, 134–136
Research
  advances in, x
  areas for, 30
  challenges for, 29–30, 38
  injury definitions' effect on, 28
  innovative approaches to, 30–37
  Sports as a Laboratory Assessment
    Model application. *See* Sports as
    a Laboratory Assessment Model
Response expectation theory, 175
Return to work, 130
Rostral brainstem, 46
Rotational forces, 50–51

S-100B, 58–60
Screening
  cognitive functioning, 97–99
  concussion, 98f, 99
  by emergency management services,
    183
  indications for, 24b
Second impact syndrome, 133
Severe traumatic brain injury,
    14t–15t
Severity of injury. *See* Injury severity
Shear stress, 48–49
Simple concussion, 26b
Single-photon-emission computed
    tomography, 69–70
Societal effects, 9–10, 129
Socioeconomic status, 5
Sodium-potassium pump, 55
Somatization, 170
Somatoform disorders, 170
Sport-related concussion
  amnesia after, 120
  cognitive functioning affected by,
    116–117
  continuity of care for, 34–35
  definitions of, 21, 24b–26b
  in football, 48
  functional magnetic resonance
    imaging studies, 68
  impact force, 50
  incidence of, 31–32
  long-term risks, 136–138
  loss of consciousness after, 120
  magnitude of, 50
  mild cognitive impairment risks,
    136–137
  NCAA Concussion Study,
    87–89
  neuropsychological recovery after,
    115–117
  recurrent, 133–136
  research models for, 30–37
  risk period for, 32
  studies of, 48
  symptoms of, 93
Sports
  football. *See* Football
  incidence in, 31–32

About the Author

Dr. Michael McCrea is the Executive Director of the ProHealth Care Neuroscience Center based in suburban Milwaukee, Wisconsin. Dr. McCrea is a board-certified clinical neuropsychologist and has headed the Neuropsychology Service at Waukesha Memorial Hospital since 1996. He earned his doctoral degree from the University of Wisconsin-Milwaukee, completed his clinical training in neuropsychology at Vanderbilt University School of Medicine, and did a postdoctoral fellowship at Northwestern University Medical School. An active researcher in the neurosciences, Dr. McCrea has published numerous scientific publications and book chapters, and has given national and international lectures on the topic of traumatic brain injury.